A FORTY-YEAR RETROSPECTIVE OF PRESIDENT NIXON'S COMMITTEE ON HEALTH EDUCATION

A Whistle-Blower's Diary

JOY GARRISON CAUFFMAN
AND RONALD L. LINDER

iUniverse, LLC.
Bloomington

A FORTY-YEAR RETROSPECTIVE OF PRESIDENT NIXON'S COMMITTEE ON HEALTH EDUCATION A WHISTLE-BLOWER'S DIARY

iUniverse books may be ordered through booksellers or by contacting:

iUniverse
1663 Liberty Drive
Bloomington, IN 47403
www.iuniverse.com
1-800-Authors (1-800-288-4677)

Because of the dynamic nature of the Internet, any web addresses or links contained in this book may have changed since publication and may no longer be valid. The views expressed in this work are solely those of the author and do not necessarily reflect the views of the publisher, and the publisher hereby disclaims any responsibility for them.

Any people depicted in stock imagery provided by Thinkstock are models, and such images are being used for illustrative purposes only.

Certain stock imagery © Thinkstock.

ISBN: 978-1-4759-9583-1 (sc)
ISBN: 978-1-4759-9584-8 (hc)
ISBN: 978-1-4759-9585-5 (e)

Library of Congress Control Number: 2013911090

Printed in the United States of America.

iUniverse rev. date: 7/26/2013

To the future of health education

CONTENTS

PREFACE

Over the past sixty-one years, Joy Garrison Cauffman has provided leadership throughout the world in health education. She started her teaching career in a junior and senior high school in Ohio, upon completing her BS in education at Ohio State University. During several years of teaching in public and private schools, she completed her MA in physical education and subsequently her PhD in health education and health-care administration at Ohio State University. After several years on the public health faculty at UCLA, she accepted an invitation from USC School of Medicine to join the faculty and the task force during the Watts Riots.

Dr. Cauffman was the first woman to serve as president of the USC Medical Faculty Assembly and receive a full professorship, on the tenure track, in the Department of Family Medicine at USC. In 1995, she was inducted into the State of Ohio Women's Hall of Fame for her extraordinary accomplishments as an international lecturer and advisor to three United States presidents on health education and physical fitness.

Although her dissent on President Nixon's Committee on Health Education created several years of difficult times, in 1999, she was inducted into the College of Education and Human Ecology Hall of Fame at Ohio State University for her lifetime contributions as a national and international model for all others in the field. Her published results in prominent peer-reviewed journals changed physicians' screening advice for colon cancer worldwide.

During her sabbatical from USC in 1993, she conducted a continuing medical education study, "Effects of Continuing Medical Education Interventions on Physician Performance and Patient Health Care Outcomes: A Ten-Year International Study of Randomized Controlled Trials with Family Physicians or General Practitioners." The outcomes of this study resulted in invitations from seven countries to present the knowledge base on the effectiveness of continuing education for primary care physicians.

Dr. Cauffman's vision of a coalition became a reality in 1971. She envisioned the benefits and power of collaboration among the various national professional organizations with interest in health education. She was elected a Fellow by four of the eight coalition organizations and received the coalition's "Distinguished Service Award" in addition to Eta Sigma Gamma's "Distinguished Writer's Award" for her monograph, "A History of the Coalition of National Health Education Organizations: Its First Ten Years and Future Directions" in 1984.

As an honors student, Ronald L. Linder graduated with BA and MS degrees in health education from the University of Washington, an EdD in health education from the University of Oregon, and a National Science Foundation postdoctoral fellowship in research at Stanford University. He started his teaching career at Alaska Methodist University at twenty-three years of age.

He was a fellow of the American School Health Association at twenty-six. After chairing the Teaching Credential and Graduate Programs in health education at San Francisco State University for four years, he joined Dr. Joy Cauffman on the SEARCH: A Link to Services project at USC School of Medicine in 1974. He later coordinated the National Science Foundation's Biomedical Interdisciplinary Curriculum Project for four years, prior to his administrative and faculty positions in public health, medicine, and education at UCLA in 1978. His background in psychoactive drug abuse research led to coauthoring the first book on PCP abuse; *PCP: The Devil's Dust— Recognition, Management, and Prevention of Phencyclidine Abuse* was published in 1981. He has written articles in professional journals, monographs, and was awarded a million-dollar grant to train twelve thousand human service providers on PCP abuse throughout the state of California. He served as expert witness on many homicide and DUI cases related to PCP abuse during the past thirty years.

After several years teaching, administrating postgraduate medical education, consulting, and acting as the principal investigator on several UCLA training grants; he became director of education at the Hospital Satellite Network and subsequently was president of American Medical Productions, winner of Telly Awards for medical television. Dr. Linder became Regional Liaison Officer, Veterans Health Administration Western Region for the Ambulatory Care and Education Initiative for five years. He created the Ambulatory Care Consultation and Education Support Services (ACCESS) program used to evaluate and transition selected inpatient to outpatient care.

In 1999, he coauthored *Home Health Telecommunications*. A few years later, he established two substance abuse treatment programs for the underserved in Los Angeles. Dr. Linder has received numerous awards and recognitions for his work, including a "Medical Aspects of Nuclear Weapons and Nuclear War" symposium in 1981, which contributed to the International Physicians for the Prevention of Nuclear War receiving the Nobel Prize for Peace in 1985.

INTRODUCTION

Shortly after moving into a townhouse east of Los Angeles in 1988, I learned that Dr. Ron Linder's in-laws were my next-door neighbors. What were the chances of that happening within a surrounding population of millions of people? Ultimately, I didn't believe it was just chance; it was meant to be. Ron worked for me thirty-seven years ago on the SEARCH project, which was during my dissent on President Nixon's Committee on Health Education. My dissent identified the activities of a bogus presidential committee that was used to promote legislation that maintained the powers that be in America's health-care system.

Ron and I spent several months documenting daily events and retaliations against me as a result of my dissent as a member of President Nixon's committee. Since we were ultimately discovered documenting everything and possibly sharing it with others as a diary, it didn't take long for Ron to also be threatened. When he and his fiancée were at a taping of a television show in December 1974, his car, parked in a metered space on the street, was crushed from both ends, like an accordion.

When the police arrived, they asked, "What are you doing? This is usually related to organized crime."

Ron called a close friend in law enforcement. His friend said, "Stop what you are doing and get out of Los Angeles."

We learned several years later that Nixon's "Plumbers" were in Los Angeles for the Ellsberg break-in during the time of Ron's car incident. I doubt we will ever know for sure.

Also, my husband, Charles E. Cauffman, a Naval Academy Graduate, Blue Angel pilot, test pilot, and astronaut, upon retirement was encouraged to apply for director of Los Angeles International Airport. Although he was told that the position would definitely be his, it didn't happen. In retrospect, I now believe it was quite possible that I triggered his being ultimately turned down, since his application for the job was after my dissent. We also discovered that our home telephones were being tapped.

Although I continued documenting, Ron immediately stopped and quickly moved out of Los Angeles to coordinate a National Science Foundation (NSF) project at the University of California at Berkeley. We have discovered that the late Samuel Sherman, MD, director of the Regional Medical Program (changed to The Health Systems Management Corporation in 1976), under which the NSF project was funded, was instrumental in getting Ron out of Los Angeles.

Dr. Sherman, past president of the California Medical Association, was also responsible in moving Ron back to Los Angeles as associate director of health sciences, UCLA Extension and on faculty in the Schools of Public Health, Medicine, and Education at the completion of the NSF project.

The late Dr. Martin Schickman, who hired Ron at UCLA, claimed that the letter of recommendation from Dr. Sherman was the most impressive he had ever seen. Dr. Sherman, close to the leaders of the President's Committee, was appointed to the board of directors of the National Center for Health Education, the major recommendation of the President's Committee on Health Education. Ron now believes he was being rewarded for leaving town and no longer communicating with me.

Over the past twenty-three years of living here, I have waved to Ron from my home on several occasions when he was visiting his in-laws. During the past thirty-seven years, we have never talked about those days of documenting my dissent, out of fear of retaliation.

Given current federal commitments to initiate national health-care reform and the related reasons for my dissent, a current democratic president, the death of half of the members of the committee, and the need to share with others the impact of my dissent on all of our lives, Ron called me and requested a meeting to consider returning to where we left off nearly forty years earlier. Over the years, we have not been able to close this door due to fear. After what we have been through, it is time to share the reasons for my dissent to promote the commitment of others to preserve our democracy through the freedom of speech without retaliation. My wish at eighty-six years, having spent the balance of my life trying to regain my identity, is that others who know my story will become advocates of the right to dissent and protect those who do. It is a critical part of our freedom, democracy, and survival, in addition to the future of the coalition, which I created, of national health-education organizations.

Our first goal was to locate the boxes of documentation that were stored in my garage for nearly forty years. After Ron's arrival and a brief conversation about the past thirty-eight years, we went into the garage and started searching for the boxes. We were quite excited to discover a large inventory of fifty-three boxes, placed twenty-three years ago under a heavy plastic sheet, in storage cabinets on the back wall between the garage and the house. From the two rows of boxes on the shelves, Ron randomly picked one from the center to see if we were on the right track. The first box contained two large notebooks and related materials with written documentation on my dissent from 1973 to 1974. Fortunately, each box had been sealed, and the contents appeared to be in extremely good condition. We ultimately retrieved nine boxes that contained fifteen four-inch notebooks filled with information on the history of my work on the committee. Each notebook contained a written description of activities by day and month, very much like a diary, including related documents. After a quick examination of the notebooks, we recognized several titles from our original outline.

We realized immediately that it would take many hours to read through each notebook, with an average of two to three hundred pages of documentation, including summaries of activities, minutes from meetings, phone conversations, letters and memos, reports, notices, and interpretations of events leading to my dissent.

After briefly looking through several notebooks, we decided our first step would be to review all the material in detail and then decide how best to organize it to share with others. Ron was my official alternate on President Nixon's committee and had attended one of my meetings in Chicago, which contributed to the completion of this book. We decided to structure the content of the notebooks as a retrospective with flashback scenarios, current remarks, and subsequent interpretations.

Health education, the mission of President Nixon's committee, played a major role in the future of health care in 1972, as it does today. Without educating people on how to live in good health, to reach their potentials, maintain quality of life, prevent many diseases, and access proper health-related resources, we will never achieve our goals in health-care reform. Without ongoing health education of both children and adults, the cost of health care will continue to rise beyond our ability to ever provide proper care for the masses, including the rapidly growing population of older Americans.

In addition to presenting essential background for interpreting the reasons for my dissent, Dr. Linder and I will be sharing our current outlooks on the documentation of the past, which should reveal the impact of my actions forty years ago on the future of health education in America.

How did I get into this challenging mess, leading to many years of retribution for my doing the right thing as a member of President Nixon's Committee on Health Education? I became a whistle-blower. Many on Nixon's team did not want that whistle to blow out of fear it would add yet another negative incident to Nixon's reputation, which already included the Pentagon Papers and Watergate. The consequences of my dissent appeared to have more strings attached than I ever anticipated. My story became the biggest single threat to the President's Committee leaders, and they wanted to keep the politics of truth hidden. It took courage, but I know I did the right thing. I'm glad I did, and I hope I've set an example for others to follow. The ultimate price to be paid by all is the result of not dissenting. Our survival requires it. The impact of politics on the future of health education is demonstrated throughout this book. I hope my diary of events will enable you to better understand what actually happened and why it happened—an important lesson for all of us. There must be a nonpartisan approach to mending fences and reconciling the conflicts that continue to impede the potential benefits of health education to Americans.

A Forty-Year Retrospective of President Nixon's Committee on Health Education is the inside truth of my dissent. A special thanks to Becky Smith, Kerry Redican, Mark Temple, and Larry Olsen, true leaders in our field, for their support in getting our story to you.

PART 1

PRESIDENT NIXON'S COMMITTEE ON HEALTH EDUCATION

On February 18, 1971, President Richard M. Nixon presented his "Health Message to Congress."

> In the last twelve months alone, America's medical bill went up 11 percent, from $63 to $70 billion. In the last ten years, it has climbed 170 percent, from the $26 billion level in 1960. Then we were spending 5.3 percent of our gross national product on health; today we devote 7 percent of our gross national product on health expenditures ... We spend vast sums to treat illnesses and accidents that could be avoided for a fraction of those expenditures. We focus our attention on making people well rather than keeping people well, and—as a result—both our health and our pocketbooks are poorer. A new national health strategy should assign a much higher priority to the work of prevention.

The president highlighted measures to be taken "against the long-range causes of illnesses and accidents." One of these measures was health education.

> In the final analysis, each individual bears the major responsibility for his own health. Unfortunately, too many of us fail to meet that responsibility. Too many Americans eat too much, drink too much, work too hard, and exercise too little. Too many are careless drivers.
>
> These are personal questions, to be sure, but they are also public questions. For the whole society has a stake in the health of the individual. Ultimately, everyone shares in the cost of his illnesses or accidents. Through tax payments and through insurance premiums, the careful subsidize the careless, the nonsmokers subside those who smoke, the physically fit subsidize the ignorant and vulnerable.
>
> It is in the interest of our entire country, therefore, to educate and encourage each of our citizens to develop sensible health practices. Yet we have given remarkably little attention to the health education of our people. Most of our current efforts in this area are fragmented and haphazard—a public service advertisement one week, a newspaper article another, a short lecture now and then from the doctor. There is no national instrument, no central force to stimulate and coordinate a comprehensive health education program.
>
> I have therefore been working to create such an instrument. It will be called the National Health Education Foundation. It will be a private, nonprofit group that will receive no federal money. Its membership will include representatives of business, labor, the medical profession, the insurance industry,

health and welfare organizations, and various governmental units. Leaders from these fields have already agreed to proceed with such an organization and are well on the way toward reaching an initial goal of $1 million in pledges for its budget. This independent project will be complemented by other federal efforts to promote health education.

At the same time President Nixon presented his message to Congress, the American Association for Health, Physical Education, and Recreation (AAHPER), School Health Division (an affiliate of the National Education Association, the largest professional organization in the world) was reevaluating its role in national health-education affairs. On April 6, 1971, the division council took action to explore the feasibility of a federation of national health-education organizations. The concept of the feasibility study was subsequently approved through consensus of the AAHPER board of directors. My professional colleagues requested that I assume the leadership role in conducting the feasibility study. After careful consideration, I accepted the challenge.

THE NEENAH 8

With the assistance of my peers, criteria were established for selecting national organizations to participate in the study and raise funds to underwrite the costs for a national conference. Eight national organizations with active health-education programs and health-educator memberships accepted the invitation to participate in the study:

- Health Education Section, American College Health Association
- School Health Division, American Association for Health, Physical Education, and Recreation

- Public Health Education Section, American Public Health Association
- School Health Section, American Public Health Association
- American School Health Association
- Conference of State and Territorial Directors of Public Health Education
- Society of State Directors of Health, Physical Education, and Recreation
- Society of Public Health Educators, Inc.

The first mini conference, hosted by Kimberly-Clark Corporation, was held in Neenah, Wisconsin, on May 9–11, 1971. The conference was devoted to exploring the feasibility of a federation, identifying and prioritizing common interests and concerns, considering points of view toward forming a federation, describing the structure of a coalition, and planning for a follow-up conference.

The conference was referred to as the "Neenah 8," which was interlaced with President Nixon's Health Message to Congress. The conference was in line with changing patterns in consumer health education and a logical part of the evolution of the health-education profession. In the past fifty years, health education has achieved academic and professional status in more than one hundred higher education institutions throughout the United States. The following excerpt is from the conference proceedings:

> Public and school health educators now believe that the profession must achieve greater autonomy for self-direction through some type of an amalgamation of effort. We must cooperatively plan comprehensive health education programs, eliminating both fragmentation and duplication ... This can be achieved only when we unify our efforts and speak out as one voice.

The Neenah 8 was established to combine our efforts to espouse the cause of organized health education, since others could take our place. Advertising and marketing are usually the primary goals of health commercials. The promotion of prescription drugs on national television and the Internet lacks true educational value at a time when most people lack the basic school health education to interpret such information. Yet the interest in health and medicine has grown rapidly, as evidenced by the vast number of current daytime and primetime television shows, from *Dr. Oz,* and *The Doctors* to *ER* and *Grey's Anatomy.* Also, the growing need and desire for consumer health information and education today is evidenced by the rapid expansion of health topics on cable television and the Internet, which are vital options for future delivery of health information and education, a critical part of health-care reform.

President Nixon's Health Message to Congress, the first Neenah conference, and the creation of the nation's first presidential Committee on Health Education represented major events—for the first time in history—to take comprehensive health education to the people. This was exciting. Unfortunately, President Nixon's underlying motives were hidden behind the mask of well-written recommendations in his message to Congress and the members of the Committee on Health Education.

APPOINTMENT TO THE PRESIDENT'S COMMITTEE

During 1970–1972, I was serving as the vice president for school health of AAHPER. At this time, Laura Mae Brown, president of AAHPER, had been asked by Secretary Elliot Richardson to recommend, on behalf of the association, the names of individuals who might effectively serve as members of President Nixon's Committee on Health Education.

While attending the AAHPER National Convention in Detroit in April 1972, Brown stopped me in the hall and said, "Joy, I sent a letter to President Nixon recommending you represent school health on his health-education committee. You are likely to receive the appointment, and I know you will do an outstanding job."

Laura Mae Brown deeply moved me with her statement, since she and I were often on opposite sides on certain professional issues discussed within the association. She was special.

During the next six months, I did not receive any official information about the President's Committee on Health Education, although it was a hot topic of conversation at the Neenah 8 meeting in Wisconsin in May 1971.

In the fall, I attended the Annual American Public Health Association meeting in Minneapolis, during which President Nixon's newly created Committee on Health Education warranted a special session. At the time, there were only fourteen members on the committee. No person specifically represented school health education. Also, no women, representatives from rural America, or Spanish-speaking Americans were on the current roster. I quickly learned that there was much dissatisfaction within the ranks.

Once it had been confirmed that the President's Committee on Health Education had no representation from professionals in the field of health education, I was motivated to take on the task of getting myself on the committee or someone else qualified and willing to take on the challenge.

As acting coordinator of the new tenuously coalesced group of national health-education organizations, I felt compelled to bring needed representation from health education to the unbalanced presidential committee. I was going directly from Minneapolis to Washington, DC, on professional business. Since I am not a stranger at our nation's capital, perhaps I could find someone who might help me promote representation on the committee.

While in Washington, I met with Carl A. Troester Jr., the executive secretary of AAHPER. I said, "Our people believe we have a real crisis. There are no school health educators on President Nixon's Committee on Health Education, which was just unveiled in Minneapolis. Do you have any suggestions on how we still might get representation on the committee?"

He said, "Joy, AAHPER officially supported your appointment to the committee. A letter of recommendation, along with your biographical statement, was sent to President Nixon. We followed up by phone several times. Support phone calls also were made from our colleagues in the National Education Association. It seems inconceivable that school health would not be represented. Could your congressman help?"

"Thank you. Let me think about that approach."

In my hotel room, I thought about this option, but I decided not to contact my local congressman, Alphonzo Bell. I knew several other congressmen better; one in particular had been an elementary-school classmate of mine and a lifelong friend. We were both raised in the little rural town of Blanchester, Ohio. We once competed in the same arithmetic and spelling bees and often saw each other in the same swimming holes. On one occasion, we were fined for swimming together off an island in Lake Cowan.

Two days later, I had lunch with Congressman Clarence J. Brown Jr. at the House of Representatives Dining Room in the Cannon Building. His nickname was Buddy. He was a big man, over six feet in height and weighing over two hundred pounds. He was of the "Brown Dynasty" among Ohio Republications, dating back to the 1920s, when his father Clarence J. Brown Sr. was a congressman from Ohio.

I said, "I'm deeply concerned about what is happening nationally. How can President Nixon appoint a committee on health education without any representation from school health? Ninety percent of the health educators in this nation are teaching in school health. Can you imagine a study on medical education without representation from the largest professional group of physicians?"

"Absolutely not. What is the charge to the committee?"

I paraphrased the charge for Buddy.

"Yes," he replied. "School health educators must be represented."

I said, "There are several outstanding leaders throughout the nation who I am certain were recommended for membership on the committee."

"Joy, is that the committee brochure? May I see it?'

"Yes. There are already representatives on the committee from the University of Michigan and the AMA."

"Weren't you recommended for the committee?"

"Yes, by the AAHPER-NEA. Secretary Elliot Richardson invited the association to suggest nominees for the committee."

"Well then, let's find out what happened to your recommendation. Finish your coffee while I make a call."

Brown knew of my lifelong commitment to national health-education affairs, my leadership role in the AAHPER-NEA, as well as at state and regional affiliates, over the years and of my more recent effort to bring unity to several professional health-education organizations through a coalition.

Putting down his phone, Brown said, "I have some good news. I contacted William E. Timmons, head of the Congressional Relations Team and assistant to the president for legislative affairs. He was a close friend of Dad's when he was in Congress. Usually, their appointments are made by H. R. Haldeman, assistant to the president, and in charge of White House operations. You will be in the city tomorrow, won't you?"

"Yes, I will be here through Sunday."

"Give me your local phone number before you leave. If you have time this evening, you should prepare a brief vitae."

"I'll go back to the hotel now and prepare the vitae."

Early the next morning, an AAHPER secretary prepared my vitae.

Shortly after nine o'clock, I received a phone call from Robert Laur, member of the staff council on the President's Committee, Department of Health Education and Welfare, who wanted me to come to his office. I immediately caught a cab, and I was ushered into his office before ten. He interviewed me about my professional work in health education. The vitae I had prepared the night before served as an outline for our discussion.

At the conclusion of the interview, we talked about a mutual colleague, Dr. Roger O. Egeberg. In addition to several leadership positions in California, Roger became dean of the school of medicine at USC from 1994 to 1996. During that time, I was a member of his task force that went into the Watts area, during the riots in 1992, to offer health-care services and establish a neighborhood health center.

In 1969, as a democrat, Roger was Nixon's second choice for assistant secretary of health and scientific affairs, HEW, the number-one health position in the nation. In 1971, Dr. Egeberg was given three prestigious positions within the Nixon Administration.

Mr. Laur said, "Before you leave, I would also like to have Judith Moore interview you."

Moore was a research assistant in the office of assistant secretary of planning and research, HEW. We went into another conference room, and I was queried again about my professional work. I learned later that Moore was serving as a HEW staff liaison to the President's Committee on Health Education. At the conclusion of the interviews, no commitments were made. I was merely thanked for my time.

Before returning to the West Coast, I spent a couple of days in Blanchester with my dad. These brief visits with my dad and my cherished friends always served as a tonic. I knew almost everyone living in the town. As a teenager, I had taken the local census during the summer to determine how many students would be expected to attend school in the fall.

Upon returning to my office at the USC School of Medicine, I had a phone message indicating Timmons had called from the White House and I was to return his call ASAP.

He said, "Our records show school health was not appropriately represented on the committee. Your recommendations, interviews, and security check are all in order. I am pleased to announce on behalf of President Nixon that you have been appointed to his Committee on Health Education to represent the school health sector. You will be hearing from Victor Weingarten, director of the committee, this week."

I conveyed my deepest appreciation to Timmons, but he made it clear that Congressman Brown had made the appointment possible.

If I knew then what I know now, this appointment would have had the opposite impact on my emotions. In my state of "pride," I had no idea that this was the beginning of a long-standing nightmare. Interestingly, two unrelated individuals by the name of Brown made my appointment possible. I guess, once again, it was meant to be.

Among several letters of congratulations, I received:

> It is with great pleasure that I congratulate you upon your recent appointment to serve on President Nixon's Committee on Health Education. We are proud that you have received this opportunity to continue your fine work in the area of community medicine and public health. Your participation on this committee should contribute much to the present effort to solve many of the nation's problems. You and the committee have my best wishes for the success of this significant endeavor.
>
> John E. Hubbard
> President
> University of Southern California
>
> Congratulations on your presidential appointment. We are proud of you. Kindest regards.
>
> Franz K. Bauer, MD
> Dean
> School of Medicine
> University of Southern California

Congratulations on the appointment. It is a distinct
honor for both you and our institution.

Paul Wehrle, MD
Chairman
Department of Pediatrics
School of Medicine
University of Southern California

At the time of my appointment to Nixon's committee, I was an
associate professor in the School of Medicine at USC. I had two
academic appointments: community medicine and public health,
and pediatrics. I reported to Dr. Wehrle in pediatrics and Dr. Mazur
in community medicine and public health. Dr. Mazur had been a
close friend of Dr. Egeberg, who played a major role in my initial
appointment to USC.

PART 2

THE BOGUS COMMITTEE

Have you ever wondered what it would be like to serve as a member of a presidential committee? On October 20, 1971, I was appointed anchorwoman to President Richard M. Nixon's Committee on Health Education, lodged in the domestic council under John D. Ehrlichman. This presidential committee was the first on health education in the history of our nation. The inside story of this committee's activities and the ultimate release of its final report constitutes a political tragedy alongside the Watergate incident.

The charge given the committee by President Nixon was exceptionally sound. After describing the status of health education in the United States, he defined the need for health-education programs, established goals for a comprehensive nationwide effort to raise the level of "health consumer citizenship," and proposed the establishment of a National Health Foundation to carry the torch of change by implementing the committee's recommendations. We were very impressed and looked forward to great outcomes from the committee's efforts.

As time passed, many of us became disillusioned by extremely slow progress and false democratic processes. When it came time to cast our votes on the final report, the air was filled with promises, bribes, and threats of retaliation if we voted against it.

Activities involving the White House and committee leaders highly justified my dissent. The influence of committee leaders and certain corporate giants carried the goals from within the White House to a final committee report that enabled President Nixon and his men to initiate legislation that maintained the powers that be within the health-care industry. Given that the formulation of the report was at the discretion of the committee leaders, I had only two options: to approve the report or provide a statement of dissent.

In the fall of 1972, the final committee report was delivered to Secretary Elliot L. Richardson and was subsequently impounded. I started to be retaliated against for my dissent. In an effort to ensure the inclusion of my dissent in the printed report and to protect my federally funded research project (SEARCH), I revisited the White House. I met with Patrick Buchanan and James Cavanaugh.

Cavanaugh said, "Dr. Cauffman, if you submit your dissent for publication, I can lift this phone and have your grant terminated."

Unfortunately, I would not really know if this would actually happen until later, which it did.

For several months, only those in the inner circle knew of the exact whereabouts of the report. The contents were leaked to the press, radio, and television. In April 1973, nationwide coverage of the report was presented on the telecast *What You Don't Know Will Kill You*. At this time of public awareness, the complete truth was denied.

The only committee members and staff participating on the televised panel were those who supported the report. Since Joseph Beirne and I were dissenters in the final report, we were not invited to participate in the telecast.

On September 25, 1973, the report was officially received by President Nixon in a White House Press Conference and referred back to the Department of Health, Education, and Welfare for further study. The president then dismissed the committee members, and another presidential committee went into the historical records. Unfortunately, the committee's only legacy was a blue-covered bogus report. It revealed that the committee had made a mockery of the democratic process.

Ultimately, the report served as the basis for federal legislation that was passed into law, creating the force necessary to launch the first "National Center for Health Education" in the United States. The first task of the center was to undo much of the work of the committee and integrate the leadership, research, and experience of the true professionals in health education.

The waves of the Watergate and Ellsberg break-ins left their stains on the committee report and those surrounding its creation.

LATE START AND EARLY DELAY

OCTOBER 25, 1971

A letter from Weingarten asking me to join the President's Committee on Health Education finally reached my desk. He said that he had been authorized by the White House to extend the invitation. His letter contained two immediate assignments:

> The first would be to help plan our regional meeting in Los Angeles on Thursday, January 20. To do this, we would like you and Dr. Alfred Haynes, who is at the Charles Drew Medical School, to meet the initiative in bringing together a list of representative persons from both the public and private sector, as well as the non-establishment sector, who could help us determine who should be invited to testify at our January meeting, it would be very helpful … The second assignment would be to serve on the education sub-committee, which is headed by Scott Simonds, who I believe you know.

I responded to Weingarten's letter the following day, indicating that I was delighted to accept the invitation to serve on the President's

Committee. Further, I said, "I understood the intent of the two assignments and would rapidly move forward."

At the time I was appointed, the committee had been in operation for forty-two days. Although I had a late start, I did the necessary homework to catch up. One meeting had already been held in Washington during which committee members met the president and had their pictures taken.

The minutes of the first meeting of the committee held on September 14, 1971, included:

> It was agreed that the committee was deficient in not having women representatives. It was agreed that a least two would be invited to serve, and that this would be done within the next few days.

By the time I was appointed to the committee, two other women, Ella Louise Strother, president of the Provident Comprehensive Neighborhood Health Council in Baltimore, and Peggy Wright Wood, director of public social work for the Onondaga County Department of Health in Syracuse, New York, were added to the committee. I was the committee's third woman and the first and only white woman as the anchorperson. Neither Strother nor Wood, both black, were school health educators nor did they represent Spanish-speaking or rural Americans, which was a deep concern expressed by those in attendance at the APHA Conference in Minneapolis.

According to Popper's book, *The President's Commissions: How Do They Work? How Could They Work Better?*, women are underrepresented on presidential commissions. However, since two women on this committee were black, they surprisingly had better representation than white women did, although there was no Spanish-speaking representation. (In the appendix, refer to the committee's final report for information on all committee members.)

The minutes from the September meeting reported that President Nixon:

Emphasized his conviction that he was eager to have the committee explore the feasibility of creating a National Health Education Foundation, which would place major reliance upon the involvement of the private sector. He spoke of the contribution government at all levels could and should make to the effort to explore greater citizen responsibility in health matters. He said, however, that bureaucracies, no matter how efficient, did have a tendency to become stultified. He expressed the belief that the private sector could provide more creative approaches to this vital public problem. Emphasis on what a citizen could do to enhance his own health would, in the long run, make an important contribution to the nation's well-being.

Secretary Richardson, ex officio member of the President's Committee, and Dr. Merlin K. Duval Jr., assistant secretary for health affairs, Department of Health, Education, and Welfare, planned to be available to the committee at all times during its work.

The minutes from the first committee meeting revealed:

1. Walter J. McNerney, vice chairman of the committee, was president of the Blue Cross Association and president-elect of the National Health Council (NHC). He held a strategic position within the council and the committee. Earlier, McNerney had chaired the Task Force on Medicaid and Related Programs for the DHEW, under Secretary Finch. Once again, I found myself going back and forth between the committee minutes and my files. I looked under Blue Cross in my newspaper clippings. According to the Organization for Healthcare Reform (OFHR), Newsletter, April 9, 1971, issue, the Nixon Administration's national health insurance plan rested entirely on extending private

(Blue Cross and Blue Shield) and other commercial insurance companies. McNerney had admitted in a debate with Senator Edward M. Kennedy that "most of Blue Cross's 96 million subscribers can't afford the maximum benefits available." Senator Edward M. Kennedy (D-Mass.), Senator Thomas F. Eagleton (D-Mo.), and Senator Philip A. Hart (D-Mich.) claimed that "Blue Cross and Blue Shield had outlived their usefulness and questioned their ability to do the job any better in the future than they have done in the past." In the next issue, May 7, 1971, of the OFHR Newsletter, Kennedy further questioned placing a national health insurance system "in the hands of a demonstrably high-cost industry." These editorials provided an interesting backdrop to McNerney's appointment as vice chairman of the committee. If Blue Cross and Blue Shield had outlived their usefulness in the private health insurance industry, were they now seeking a new leadership role in health education?

2. "A budget of $142,000 was approved, although at the present time only $100,000 is committed. Hope was expressed that the private insurance companies and national Blue Cross, which had each agreed to contribute $50,000, would reconsider their commitment to meet the increased budget. Mr. Wilson expressed the view that the committee's work should not be impaired by lack of funds."

3. "James Cavanaugh was a White House representative to the committee." Also, he was deputy assistant secretary (regional activities and intergovernmental affairs), HEW and liaison from HEW to the President's Committee on Health Education.

4. "The committee's charge was distributed and approved." It was so well articulated and carefully designed to serve the American people. Also, it warranted a final report that reflected the true outcomes of the President's Committee, which were presented under the headings of supplementary statements (8) and dissents (2). Half of the committee members either wrote a supplementary statement or dissent to be published in the final report.

5. Weingarten "reported that the NHC had set aside a major portion of its National Health Forum in New Orleans, on March 21–22, for a 'preview' of the committee's findings and tentative recommendations." Interestingly, Blue Cross and other national insurance companies had contributed to the President's Committee on Health Education. The funds were managed by the NHC, which is under incoming Blue Cross leadership, and the committee's findings and recommendations will be presented at the forum, which is sponsored by the NHC.

Having reviewed the minutes from the first committee meeting, I got the picture.

SUBCOMMITTEE ON EDUCATION FORMED

A letter from Scott Simonds did not state the mission of the subcommittee. However, he did say that the subcommittee would initiate its work with an exploratory meeting, including a small guest group of expert health educators. This session was to be convened in Washington immediately prior to the November meeting of the full committee.

I was unable to contact Haynes to make plans for the Los Angeles Planning Committee meeting, as requested by Weingarten. Time was running out. Based on the criteria provided by Weingarten, I selected the members of the Los Angeles Regional Planning Committee, with the exception of political appointments from New York.

NOVEMBER 11, 1971

The Los Angeles Regional Planning Committee meeting was held at the Century Plaza Hotel in Century City. Before the meeting, I met Weingarten for the first time in the hotel lobby. We shook hands, exchanged greetings, and darted off to the coffee shop. Weingarten provided me with an update of committee activities and mapped out his strategy for the planning meeting. He was a bright and aggressive New Yorker who talked fast and didn't stop. Although I had prepared for the meeting, including the location, agenda, roster of participants, and special assistants, I submitted to Weingarten's wishes as to the actual conduct of the meeting.

Following the luncheon, Weingarten gave the important background statement regarding the President's Committee, including plans to hold regional hearings across the country. He then focused on the purpose of the Los Angeles regional hearing and the role of the group assembled. At the close of the meeting, I appointed Edward B. Johns, professor of health education, University of California, Los Angeles, as the chairperson for the local planning committee. He was the father of health education throughout the Western United States. Johns and the group proceeded to lay plans for subsequent committee meetings, preparing for the regional hearing on January 20, 1972, at the tax court in the Federal Building in downtown Los Angeles.

As I was leaving the meeting, I realized Haynes had not arrived. I wondered what had happened to him. I had left several messages for him, but I never heard back.

In just a few days, I would be off to the East Coast for a meeting of the Subcommittee on Education.

NOVEMBER 16, 1972

When I arrived at the APHER headquarters in Washington, the panel of school health consultants was already in session. There was no opportunity to get a briefing from Simonds on the format of the meeting.

We knew each other, but with the exception of the Neenah Conference, we had never worked together professionally. Simonds didn't appear too pleased with my presence.

Very quickly, the meeting became a brainstorming session in response to the request to develop a "pool of ideas" that the President's Committee could utilize in its deliberations.

Simonds assigned me the secretarial role, which I would have appreciated, if the minutes had ever been distributed. As the meeting progressed, trends in the field of education and models for health-education programs were being presented and discussed. It was apparent that Simonds, a public health educator, was seeking insight and wanted to become better acquainted with school health educators. He continually reminded everyone that school health education was not his specialty area, but they were educating him. He was very good at team building.

Once again, neither Haynes nor Shapiro was present. And Haynes lived in Los Angeles.

NOVEMBER 17, 1972

Prior to my trip to the East Coast, I had received and accepted an invitation from Joseph C. Wilson, chairman of the President's Committee and chairman of the Xerox Corporation, for cocktails and a buffet dinner at the Madison Hotel. *This is the night; I must hurry to make the party.*

When I arrived, Wilson noticed that I had brought a coat.

"Are you staying elsewhere in the city?" he asked.

"Yes, I wasn't able to get a room at the Madison."

As Wilson suggested in his letter, the party was a pleasant way for us to spend some time together. As a very gracious host, he escorted me around the room and introduced me to members of the committee and staff.

McNerney was the only person who made a flattering remark that was unexpected. He said, "You have pretty legs."

"Thank you."

I met Levitt Mendel, staff to the President's Committee and associate director of the NHC and Clarence Pearson, associate director to the committee and director for administration and planning for the Metropolitan Life Insurance Company.

Pearson said, "Joy, invite Lev to your next federation meeting."

Knowing the NHC did not meet the membership criteria, I guarded my reply. "Yes, I'll be in touch with Lev by letter."

The boys were already on the move.

Upon leaving the dinner party, Wilson remembered that I was not staying at the Madison. "Joy, I have arranged for Peter Warter on my staff to see you to your hotel. I know I would not want my wife to go out alone in the evening in Washington, DC."

I was moved by his thoughtfulness.

The next morning, the committee meeting was held at the Executive Office Building at the White House. The three new female members of the committee were introduced. Included among the twenty committee members were two ex officio members, Richardson and Richard P. McGrail, the current president of the NHC. McGrail was an attorney and had been the deputy vice president of the American Cancer Society since 1961.

Two public health educators and one school health educator—me— were members of the committee. The committee's staff was composed of six public health educators and no school health educators, yet over 90 percent of health educators throughout the United States teach in our schools. In periods of economic difficulties, the importance of saving vast sums of money through school health education becomes once again a logical alternative. Through education, we can lower the costs of many preventable health problems—and the quality of life among those who apply such education can be significantly improved. Since we know how to prevent and manage many expensive health problems better than ever before, it's time to include health education of children and adults (based on the principles of lifelong learning) as a major component in American's health-care reform.

SLUSH FUNDS PREVAIL

NOVEMBER 18, 1971

Other items on the agenda included two progress reports, sent to us before the meeting, which were now being explained more fully. The following quote from the first report caught my eye:

> At the moment, we are operating with the $142,000 budget originally approved. Of the sum, the Blues and the insurance companies have each contributed $50,000. McNerney is prepared to contribute another $21,000. Siegfried appears indifferent—if not resistant.

Charles A. Siegfried, a member of our committee, was vice chairman of the board and chairman of the executive committee of Metropolitan Life Insurance Company. It appeared from the written report and from the related dialogue that the Nixon Administration was pressuring Siegfried and Henry Smith, president of the Equitable Life Assurance Society, to contribute more funds to support the work of the committee.

As the committee's revised budget was reviewed, it appeared that a significant amount of additional funds would be forthcoming.

Among the unanswered questions: How much, by whom, and under what circumstance? The amounts discussed could vastly exceed the formal budget. I had no idea that this was the last time I would ever see the committee's budget. I was never included in any subsequent reports or formal discussions on the budget or outside funds. In light of the threats from my dissent that caused us to stop documenting, were any of these funds involved in the Watergate incident? There was a lot of speculation at that time.

Henceforth, the budget remained a secret document shared only by those of the "inner circle." A direct relationship existed between certain committee members and the funds that their employers were contributing to the committee. For example, the Blues had contributed $50,000, and were willing to provide more. At least three members of the committee—McNerney, John Alexander McMahon, a member of the board of governors and executive committee of the Blue Cross Association and the president of the American Hospital Association, and Joseph T. Painter, a member of the Medical Care Advisory Committee of the board of directors of Blue Cross/Blue Shield of Texas—were directly associated with Blue Cross operations.

Many of the committee members were appointed through recommendations of the health insurance industry. I know Haynes had close personal and professional ties with members of the Equitable Life Insurance Company. Simond's wife was a former employee of the Metropolitan Life Insurance Company and was a close friend of Pearson.

When the Neenah Conference was held in May 1971, Simonds thought he might be able to announce to the conferees that he had been appointed to the presidential committee. Several calls were made from Neenah to the Metropolitan Life Insurance Company in New York to obtain word on his appointment, but it did not happen at the time.

With respect for the six public health educators on the committee's staff, one represented the Blues, two were from the private insurance companies, two were affiliated with the NHC, and one was with a voluntary health organization.

I wondered if all presidential committees were similar. In referencing Frank Popper's *The President's Commissions,* I realized our committee was not a commission. There are differences and similarities between committees and commissions.

> Most commissions in the past have been created by
> executive order of the president and are financed by
> emergency, executive, or special projects funds, all of
> which can be expanded as the president mandates.
> When these funds are lacking, commissions can be
> created and financed by legislation, which Congress
> routinely passes at the request of the president.

Popper made no comments about companies of commission members supporting committee functions. He did claim that the amount that presidents give to commissions varied from half a million to two million dollars.

The President's Committee on Health Education initially had a budget of only $144,000, and the largest portion of this budget was donated by the insurance industry. Why didn't the funds to support the committee come from the federal government rather than the insurance industry? Why were the insurance companies hiding under the cloak of the federal government in the form of a presidential committee?

As the morning session continued, a major portion was devoted to a presentation on health education by Weingarten. I noted an immediate problem. The activities were not directly related to the objectives stated in the charge to the committee, but I held my tongue. The committee again and again faced this issue as it struggled to develop a report to the president.

The luncheon for the committee was served in the West Wing of the White House. As we strolled through the halls, we were impressed by the beautiful photographs of the First Family. H. R. Haldeman was reportedly responsible for the displays. The food at the luncheon was good but not exceptional; the beef was tough. The luncheon was a social occasion with the exception of the introduction of Kenneth R. Cole Jr., a member of the United States Domestic Council. In addition to Cavanaugh, Cole would serve as a White House liaison to the committee.

The committee's afternoon session was brief. Reports on regional hearings, the National Health Forum, and subcommittee activities were made. Weingarten announced that Painter was chairing the Professional Associations and Societies Subcommittee. He had made contacts with the AMA, the American Academy of Pediatrics, and other professional groups "whose activities might be of interest to the President's Committee." It was particularly enlightening to realize that no mention was made of the "professional associations and societies" where health education was the primary goal. Again, no reference was made to the Neenah Conference, the largest group of health educators in the country.

Special attention was given to the letter Wilson had received from President Nixon following the last full committee meeting.

> I am deeply pleased that you have accepted, as the Chairman of the President's Committee on Health Education, the challenging task of helping us to discover new ways in which our fellow citizens can become better educated and informed about their health. Our recent meeting to discuss this problem of enhanced health education was indeed encouraging, and it is particularly gratifying to know you will be participating in this project. At a time when it is essential for us to make the best possible use of our medical resources, it is all the more important that every American be fully aware of the measures he himself can take for his own well-being and personal health. Government, of course, has a part to play in preventive health maintenance, but the ultimate success of our efforts depends on the people themselves. That is why I consider the role of the committee so necessary in finding those means of reaching the people with this message. You and your colleagues have my very best wishes as you begin this

work and needless to say, I look forward to learning of
the progress you have made in the months ahead.

The letter contained important statements that the committee would review in drafting its final report to the president.

As I left the Old Executive Building, I said to Weingarten, "If there is anything I can do to further the efforts of the committee, let me know."

His secretary, who was standing by his side, said, "If you offer to help, I'm afraid you will get more than you bargained for. Vic will interpret your willingness to help in personal ways."

I didn't say anything more, and I continued on my way.

What was that all about? I'm not sure I want to know.

NOVEMBER 19, 1971

I stayed overnight in Washington and headed for Dulles Airport in the morning to return to Los Angeles. I kept reviewing the events of the past twenty-four hours. I felt compelled to share two ideas with Wilson. First, I believed we needed to establish a more direct relationship between committee activities and the charge to the committee.

Second, we needed to identify those health problems that contributed to high morbidity and mortality statistics in our nation. From the group of problems, we needed to select those that could be prevented, reduced, and/or controlled through education.

With some extra time at the airport, I decided to call Wilson. I located him in his office in New York City and shared my ideas with him.

Wilson said, "I like very much what you have suggested. They are both sound concepts."

I responded, "With your approval, I would like to develop tentative strategies for integrating these concepts into the committee's plan of action."

Wilson hesitated. "Joy, I must be honest with you—there is a problem. The public health educators on the committee and staff may oppose you."

It was interesting that he made no mention of other more powerful committee members who might oppose me.

"In spite of the potential problem you have shared with me, do I have your permission to proceed and to be heard by the full committee?"

"Absolutely. In fact, let me ask you to communicate with me by letter before the end of December. A copy of your letter to me should go to both McNerney and Weingarten. Then, you will be on the agenda for the committee's February meeting."

"Excellent," I said.

"Thanks for calling, Joy."

On the airplane, I reviewed handouts distributed at the full committee meeting. In reading the Subcommittee on Education report that Simonds had submitted, I noticed that he had not listed those subcommittee members not in attendance at the two-day meeting. Rather, he said:

> The Subcommittee on Education consists of Dr. Joy Cauffman, Dr. Irving Shapiro, Dr. Alfred Haynes, and myself. The committee has met twice, although not all committee members have been present at each session.

This was an effective cover-up for Shapiro and Haynes. Neither had attended the two subcommittee meetings. I realized that the subcommittee minutes I had recorded would merely become an internal document for the subcommittee since they were not included in the report to the full committee. I did not know at the time that the minutes from the November full committee meeting would never be distributed.

PRESIDENT'S COMMITTEE ON HOLD

NOVEMBER 22, 1971

Without warning, Wilson died of an apparent heart attack. His leadership in transforming the Haloid Corporation into the Xerox Corporation, a $1.7 billion industrial giant, was impressive. According to the *New York Times*, Wilson was lunching with Governor Nelson Rockefeller at the time of his death. Our committee activities were immediately put on hold. In response to Wilson's death, the White House asked that the work of the committee continue. My conversation just prior to his death was now lost. It would be some time before we could move ahead.

Newspaper stories reported that Wilson had chaired Governor Rockefeller's Steering Committee on Social Problems (referred to as the Rockefeller Report). I obtained a copy of the Rockefeller Report and reviewed the gallery of names in the report. I noted that, in addition to Wilson, Smith was a member of the President's Committee on Health Education. Also, the director of the Rockefeller Committee was Weingarten; McNerney was a consultant.

Without question, the President's Committee on Health Education was overrepresented by members from the state of New York. In addition, some members of the committee, who were listed as residing in other states, also had New York offices. Even more significant was the fact that so many of our committee members had served Rockefeller and had worked together previously.

What are the implications for the future?

SUBCOMMITTEE ON EDUCATION WIRED

NOVEMBER 26, 1971

I received a letter from Simonds. An enclosure contained the "Pool of Ideas" from the November 16 subcommittee meeting. He recommended that we also ask the delegates for ideas to add to our pool at the second coalition mini conference in December.

Simonds indicated that he would contact William Carlyon, delegate to the coalition from the American College Health Association and assistant director for the Department of Health Education, American Medical Association, before our next coalition meeting in order "to move ahead with college health groups," whatever that meant. He then added, "They were omitted from our consultant panel in Washington."

Simonds would have the opportunity to obtain Carlyon's input at the second coalition meeting. I wondered if there were other reasons why he was meeting independently with Carlyon and the college health group.

After reading Simond's letter, I asked, "What is the mission of the subcommittee? How can we utilize ideas if we do not know where we are going?"

While Simonds and I were in New York, we were invited to Weingarten's Uptown apartment overlooking the Hudson River for breakfast. I inadvertently learned the subcommittee had operating funds—or more specifically, Simonds had funds—for subcommittee activities.

Simonds said, "Vic, I need several thousand dollars to pay Mrs. Pauline Carlyon (William Carlyon's wife) for her subcommittee services. Can this be arranged?"

"Would the university provide in-kind support for her services?"

"No, that is not possible."

"Okay, go ahead and hire her."

At no time did Simonds bring financial issues before the subcommittee.

NOVEMBER 29, 1971

I was preparing for the second meeting of the Neenah 8 in New York, held from December 12–14, 1971. I recalled my earlier discussion with Clarence Pearson at Wilson's cocktail party, and I wrote to Mendel:

> The participating associations have restricted the list
> of conference participants for the December meeting.
> However, I would like to invite you to be our guest
> for dinner on Monday evening ... to explore areas of
> mutual interest between the National Health Council
> and the coalition.

I assumed that Pearson would quickly receive word that I had written Mendel.

DECEMBER 10, 1971

Mendel's reply to my letter, brief and to the point, arrived on December 10.

> As the President's Committee has not yet discussed
> the topic you suggest for the dinner meeting, I feel
> it would be most inappropriate for me to make any
> public statement on the subject.

Since I was not able to reach him by phone, I sent a letter indicating that there was apparently some misunderstanding. I had put Mendel to the test, but he was not willing or had been told not to discuss areas of mutual interest with coalition representatives.

COALITION POLITICS

DECEMBER 12–14, 1971

The second mini conference of the Neenah 8 was held in New York City. I continued to serve as coordinator. The most significant accomplishment of the conference was the development of a draft of a "working agreement" for a Coalition of National Health Education Organizations.

Simonds informed the group about the activities of the President's Committee on Health Education and asked for input to the subcommittee's "Pool of Ideas."

During the last day of the committee meeting, Simonds made a very important political announcement:

> I am resigning as the SOPHE delegate. The society will appoint another delegate in my place. I cannot serve both as a member of this group and as a member of the President's Committee because of a conflict of interest. I would also encourage Joy to resign for the same reason.

A lively discussion followed in reaction to Simonds's resignation, which many believed was not only unnecessary but unsound.

Simonds remained firm on his commitment and attempted to sway the group to favor my resignation as well.

I said, "I will not resign at this time. Scott should speak for himself. I consider the conflict of interest assumption not to be valid in my case."

Why would I resign at this time? The American Association for Health, Physical Education, and Recreation, School Health Division had asked me to represent them, and I was committed to doing so.

REGIONAL HEARINGS CREATE FALSE PROMISES

JANUARY 3–FEBRUARY 2, 1972

Reportedly, the primary purpose for the regional hearings was to gather information about health-education programs across the nation. Hearings were held during January 1972 in Boston, Denver, San Francisco, Houston, Pittsburgh, St. Louis, Los Angeles, and Atlanta.

Weingarten, in a memo to all members of the committee, provided two background references for review before the meetings: committee progress reports and the Louis Harris survey results, which the Blue Cross released just in time for the hearings. In fact, the official release made reference to the regional hearings and their relationship to the survey, "Harris Study Stresses Health Education Need."

McNerney spoke about our great health-education needs in the release. Actually, the findings of the survey referred to health information, not health-education needs, a confusion of terms that would later cause major problems for the committee. The process of health education involves modification of behavior, whereas the presentation of health information does not.

Since the survey was the only "needs assessment" provided, most committee members were led to believe that this was the only available information on the topic. Classical health-education literature abounds with such information. As expected, a disproportionate number of references were made to the Harris survey in newspaper stories associated with the regional hearings. Even more salient reasons for contributions by the insurance companies would most likely be revealed later.

The committee did not determine guidelines for regional hearing presentations before the fact. Therefore, there was confusion as to whether the witnesses should talk of health or of health-education needs of their constituencies. Without guidelines, the testimony could not be scientifically analyzed and utilized in developing a report for the president.

The first hearing was held in Boston, and John Knowles was the first witness. Interestingly, he also had been a consultant to Rockefeller's Steering Committee on Social Problems; in July 1972, Knowles made several statements that would have lasting influence and would be repeated in the months ahead.

Knowles said, "American doctors are uninterested in public health education because they lack training in the subject and because of a striking lack of intellectual, emotional, and economic incentive to include health education in their practice of medicine in the community." In spite of this, Knowles said, "the next major advance in the health of our citizens will come through health education and preventive medicine and not through doctors and high-cost hospitals."

The planning committee in each of the cities rolled out the red carpet. They made every effort to assure the success of the hearings by arranging official welcomes, extensive media coverage, receptions, and tours of the city. I served as a panel member at the Pittsburgh, St. Louis, and Atlanta hearings, and I was a presiding officer with Haynes at the Los Angeles hearing.

From my observations, all who wished to testify were given the opportunity to do so. (Later, I was to learn that merely testifying was useless if the information was not utilized.) Weingarten devoted much effort to placing the "big names" first on the program to ensure coverage by news media. Many of the local planners deeply resented Weingarten's last-minute intrusions in program formats after witnesses had already been assigned speaking times.

HIDDEN AGENDAS

The nature of the regional hearings is well illustrated by the Atlanta hearing, presented by Joseph A. Beirne, president of the Communications Workers of America and the other dissenter on the committee's final report. Representatives from the press were everywhere in the Peachtree Center. It was a long day under hot television lights listening to and questioning witnesses. Although the hearing was scheduled from 9 to 5, we continued until all witnesses had been heard. Many unscheduled speakers waited long hours to testify and were promised that their remarks would be given careful attention by the committee. I was impressed by the manner in which those who testified spoke out. They conveyed a personal sense of pride, conviction, and urgency in their messages.

Following the Atlanta hearing, committee members were invited to a cocktail party at the Midnight Sun, followed by dinner, dancing, and a tour of Underground Atlanta.

Dr. Richard K. Means, a professor of health education at Auburn University and a national leader in his field, presented his candid impressions of the Atlanta regional hearing at the annual meeting of the American Public Health Association, School Health Section, on November 15, 1972, in Atlantic City. Dr. Means stated:

> The following impressions, certain of them definitely personal and speculative in nature, were derived:
>
> 1. Inadequate emphasis was afforded to the significant part that schools and colleges can play in overall programs of health education. One out of thirty-one presentations at the Atlanta hearing bears witness of this fact. Further, only seven of five hundred participants at the national meeting in New Orleans had specific school health interest.
>
> 2. There is an indication that most members of the President's Committee do not actually understand health education in the true sense of the term. This was apparent in a recent article in *The Houston Post* wherein an influential committee member made the statement that "it is a 'crying shame' how little basic health data any of them received," with respect to school programs.
>
> 3. Inadequate time was allowed at the hearing for further informal testimony by those not officially invited to participate. This was due in large part to the fact that established guidelines of fifteen minutes for each presenter were not followed. This left little time for additional response.
>
> 4. It was obvious that most committee members had already developed preconceived opinions about the

deplorable state of health education in schools and colleges. Although there is agreement that programs are definitely inadequate in general, there was the impression of futility in attempting to develop and implement such programs in the future.

As the hearings concluded, it was clear that there had been many hidden agendas.

JANUARY 19, 1972

For example, at the San Francisco hearing, Weingarten announced to the *San Francisco Examiner* that the committee had a $1 million budget. This was a far cry from the $144,700 budget committee members had been informed about at the last full committee meeting. Weingarten claimed, "The US Department of Health, Education, and Welfare was footing $150,000." He added, "An estimated $700,000 would be given in the form of 'contributed time and services.'"

The Blue Cross had agreed to videotape all regional hearings for television; an edited one-hour summary following each hearing and a one-hour documentary would be constructed from the eight regional hearings.

How does this contribution work? Did the President's Committee budget in any way relate to the financing of the Watergate and Ellsberg break-ins or the Committee to Re-Elect the President? Will we ever know?

JANUARY 21, 1972

At the completion of the regional hearings, Weingarten sent me the following note:

On behalf of the President's Committee, I want to thank you for the splendid job you and your associates did in helping plan the Los Angeles regional. The list of witnesses represented a broad gauge of experience and approach, and the diversity was exactly what we wished. It is a real tribute to your planning efforts that everyone scheduled to appear did so, and that their testimony was so sharply focused and helpful.

Interestingly, although Weingarten had asked me to copreside at the Los Angeles regional hearing with Haynes, the news release did not carry such information. At the hearing, Haynes presided during the first portion of the hearing that was televised; I presided after the telecast.

FEBRUARY 4, 1972

In a letter, Simonds stated, "You were great to send the materials from the regional hearings. Pauline prepared a preliminary outline of the proposed report, which is attached for your use. It is sent to you confidentially for in no way should it be construed as the outline for the final report or circulated to others."

Pauline Carlyon had apparently been employed and had prepared a preliminary outline of the proposed report for the subcommittee.

What is the role of a member of the appointed subcommittee?

TRUE VALUES OF HEALTH EDUCATION RECOGNIZED

FEBRUARY 8, 1972

The Subcommittee on Education conducted a one-day seminar for national leaders in early childhood education, health, and parent education at the Metropolitan Life Insurance Company of New York. Organizations such as DHEW, the national PTA, and other related national associations, universities, and the President's Committee representatives—Simonds, Shapiro, Lifson, and Impellizzeri—participated in the meeting. Haynes was not at any of the subcommittee meetings, and I did not see any communications from him.

Impellizzeri had organized a great seminar. Simonds, the chair of the seminar, stated that the purpose was to "obtain advice and consultation from national leaders on needs and possibilities for health education among preschool children and their parents." It was noted in Impellizzeri's seminar minutes that the subcommittee would be preparing a report and recommendations to the full committee on the basis of this meeting, their study of the literature, and data from other sources.

The minutes also stated:

> The seminar group had explored health education that would lay foundations for the preschool child's ability to take responsibility for his own health and the health of others and the parents' ability to enhance the health of children. Examples of the kinds of health messages parents convey to their children were cited, and the scope of health-education programs were delineated. Communication channels for implementing health-education programs for preschool children and their parents were listed.

In research, the group saw a need for dissemination and interpretation of new information. They pointed out that interpreters might provide a link between researchers and implementers. The seminar group also identified impediments to effective health-education programs and proposed recommendations for the committee's consideration.

The outcomes of this seminar were similar to many others in generating outstanding insights and recommendations to bring health education to the people, both young and old. Unfortunately, most of these recommendations never got to the President's Committee.

PRESIDENT'S COMMITTEE MEETING #3

The third committee meeting was held in New York at the Metropolitan Life Insurance Company. Since our last meeting, White House staff had appointed R. Heath Larry, vice chairman of the board of directors of the US Steel Corporation, as committee chairman in place of the late Joseph C. Wilson. It came as no surprise that Larry also was a former member of Governor Rockefeller's Steering Committee on Social Problems along with the late Wilson and Smith.

Larry had gotten off to a rough start in chairing the regional hearing in Pittsburgh during January. First, he had more witnesses than available time. For example, at the Pittsburgh hearing, Robert Kaplan, professor of health education, Health Education Division at Ohio State University, wrote to me on January 12, 1972, following the hearing:

> As you know, after waiting to get on the agenda in Pittsburgh, I came close to airplane time and rushed my presentation. No doubt, the chairman's comments on hurrying were a factor too. Frankly, I found the whole thing difficult to work for since I personally doubt President Nixon's motives and sincerity. I hope the paper doesn't show my personal attitude. I plan to send the president a copy to see if he (his staff) reacts to it at all, if favorably.

On January 17, 1972, Kaplan wrote to the president, but he never heard from him or his staff.

Larry was challenged by a witness and a band of community people who accused US Steel of being a major contributor to the air pollution problem in the Pittsburg area. Panel members were given a can of "clean air" by one witness. Hostilities mounted with a heated discussion, which ended with Larry walking out of the room.

Larry's wife was hospitalized, and he was unable to attend the February committee meeting. McNerney presided in his absence and the Regional Hearing Statistical Report was given by Weingarten:

- 1,477 persons who signed the guest register
- 192 persons on regional planning councils

- 282 witnesses from forty-seven states, including Alaska, Hawaii, and Puerto Rico
- 39 additional papers submitted
- 71 hours of testimony
- 52 hours of educational television
- 6 hours of commercial radio
- commercial TV in every city
- extensive press coverage

In regard to telecasting, he explained, "All of the footage was being edited down to a ninety-minute documentary, and that additional footage would be taken at the forum in New Orleans in March. Present plans were for the National Educational Television Network to carry the documentary either the evening the committee reports to the president or the following night. Cost of this project was underwritten by the Blue Cross Association."

Weingarten also reported, "Two position papers commissioned by the committee had been completed and that other papers on motivational behavior were being prepared."

Blue Cross certainly had the opportunity to maintain its mission as the producer of these documentary segments for television. What a conflict of interest.

Simonds followed by indicating that the work of the Subcommittee on Education was progressing well, and staff support had increased. In addition to Sol Lifson, the subcommittee now had the assistance of Anne E. Impellizzeri, health-education consultant, Health and Welfare Division, Metropolitan Life Insurance Company, and Pauline M. Carlyon, a freelancer, and the wife of William Carlyon.

Simond's written report indicated that Carlyon's services "had been obtained in Michigan for an additional search of key reports and documents, for analyzing the documents and papers from the regional hearings, and for assisting with final writing of the committee report." No mention was made of any remuneration.

FEBRUARY 11–12, 1972

I arrived in Ann Arbor, Michigan, prior to the coalition mini conference. This preconference time was to be spent with Simonds and others at the University of Michigan in preparing a report for the Subcommittee on Education.

This was a difficult situation for several reasons. Foremost, there was "no clear charge or outline" for the subcommittee. Second, the other subcommittee members, Shapiro and Haynes, were not present. Third, there was never a time for Simonds and me to privately discuss some of the issues. Pauline Carlyon was always at his side. Based on Simond's earlier associations with Carlyon, it appeared that the preplanning had already taken place. Fourth, there was a push for us to prepare a preliminary draft of the report before the coalition conference, enabling us to benefit from input of the delegates. Basically, this was a sound idea, but the time period—two days—for producing even a preliminary draft of quality was too short.

Following the mini conference, I continued to contribute to the report. On February 23, Simonds sent the report to Weingarten, indicating that no recommendations had been provided at the time.

The "Preliminary Report of Findings and Recommendations" of the Subcommittee on Education (thirty-eight pages, not for duplication or distribution) contained some valuable information, delivered under the following titles:

- National and Regional Leadership for Health Education
- The Preschool Child and His Parent
- Comprehensive School Health Education Programs
- Leadership for the Development of Health Education in Schools
- Advancing the Teaching of Health in the Schools
- Health Education in Colleges and Universities

The total subcommittee appeared as authors. Of course, this was not true. It was a shocking, dishonest statement written by hired authors, not members of the President's Committee.

FEBRUARY 13–15, 1972

The Neenah 8 held its third mini conference at the University of Michigan. Momentum was building toward the formation of a Coalition of National Health Education Organizations. I anticipated the coalition would be formed before the 1972 National Health Forum, which would be sponsored in March by the National Health Council and held in New Orleans.

Seven of the eight national health-education organizations had developed position papers for the President's Committee on Health Education. These position papers were analyzed for areas of common concern and mutual interest, and they were used as a basis for formulating a "unified" position statement to be presented at the National Health Forum. Also, the specific strategy of "coalition" involvement in the National Health Forum was planned. There was general agreement that the coalition's major purposes at the forum would be to marshal support for those recommendations of the President's Committee upon which there was "coalition" consensus and to create a climate of expectation that these recommendations would be fulfilled.

Who should be the spokesperson for the coalition at the National Health Forum meeting? As coordinator of the coalition, some members felt that I should. After considerable discussion and coaching from Simonds, the group agreed that Carlyon would serve as the coalition's spokesperson at the forum. Once again, it was assumed that I could not effectively represent both the President's Committee and the coalition.

In completing our strategy for the forum, Hammond agreed to send a memo to all health educators attending the forum and to invite them to our special meeting planned for Monday evening, March 20.

During the conference program, Simonds presented the preliminary draft of the report of the Subcommittee on Education to the coalition delegates for review. He identified me as having developed parts of the report, which I could not scientifically support. This was embarrassing and caused me to lose face with the group.

Recalling my experience with Simonds at the second coalition meeting in New York City, and my more recent episode with him at the current meeting, I did not believe his intentions were honorable.

THE COALITION'S MISSION

The coalition's mission is to mobilize the resources of the health-education profession for the expansion and improvement of health education in the United States. Accordingly, the coalition will be made up of those organizations that have identifiable memberships of health educators in addition to a major commitment to health education. As the coalition addresses itself to problems and issues in health education, it will collaborate with all concerned individuals and organizations.

The specific purposes of the coalition are to

- test the viability and effectiveness of national level coordination, collaboration, and communication among the organizations involved;
- identify health-education problems of mutual concern at the national level;
- promote and take action on problems affecting the joint interests of the organizations involved.

The coalition is on a trial basis for a two-year period, principally to allow time for the participating organizations to work through operating procedures, to more clearly define the common goals that require mutual support, and to lay the foundation for more long-term organizational relationships within the coalition.

MARCH 12, 1972

The Coalition of National Health Education Organizations became a reality in March when three organizations signed the working agreement for a two-year period.

By April, all eight national professional health-education organizations in the United States had elected to become charter members of the coalition. The coalition's focus was to mobilize the resources of the health-education profession for the expansion and improvement of health education in the United States. The coalition had become the unified voice of the health-education profession, and it was striving to obtain a professional and legal identity, although "spies" among us from the National Health Council were trying to undermine our efforts. The council, under McNerney's leadership, used its giant crane in trying to pick up the coalition and place it in their backyard. As the crane's shovel came down on the coalition, several member organizations went along for the ride, but others escaped. Irreparable damage occurred to a young new viable profession.

McNerney was an opportunist. He was seeking greater political power and increased financial resources in order to serve the vested interests of the insurance industry. To achieve his purpose, McNerney would stop at nothing—including foul play, coercion, suppression, and censorship. Not until later would the American people feel the impact of the council's tyranny under his leadership. They paid heavily for health-education services as a part of their medical care insurance package.

The coalition's "working agreement" included two items related to the President's Committee on Health Education: (1) "Assessment of the Final Report of the President's Committee on Health Education" and (2) "Provision of leadership for a national audit of the final report of the President's Committee on Health Education and subsequent follow-up associated with the report. The audit, designed as an annual report, will include a conference and other related activities."

The Coalition of National Health Education Organizations is still a vibrant force in health education. Through the coalition, the profession can speak with one voice. The coalition has grown from eight member organizations to ten. Its mission is to mobilize the resources of the health-education profession in all settings.

MARCH 3, 1972

Emily M. Hammond, the director for health education, Health and Welfare Division, Metropolitan Life Insurance Company, and delegate to the coalition from the American Public Health Association, School Health Section, sent a memo to all health educators invited to attend the National Health Forum.

> For the past several months, as designated representatives of eight national professional organizations of health educators, we have been working together to explore how our organizations can cooperate to forward common concerns. We are suggesting that all health educators attending the forum have an opportunity to discuss the material to be presented and the interests of our several organizations as indicated in their statements to the President's Committee. Our group has been able to review these statements and identify a number of priorities common to all the organizations. These priorities will be considered at the meeting which will be held on Monday, March 20, from 7:30 to 8:30 p.m. in Emily Hammond's suite at the Jung Hotel. At that time, we will discuss ways in which health educators can be most effective during the forum and how we can best contribute to the implementation of the forum outcomes.

THE FINAL MEETING

MARCH 1, 1972

The fourth and final meeting of the President's Committee was held in New York in the boardroom of Equitable Life Insurance. Each cross-country trip to a full committee meeting was taking me two additional days due to travel time. These flights were often productive, since there were few interruptions.

At the meeting, Larry reported that the staff had prepared a preliminary draft of the report (the second unnumbered and undated report to my knowledge), but there had not been in many sections final agreement on the language by the executive subcommittee. I noted few differences in this draft of the report from Weingarten's earlier presentation at the November committee meeting.

The National Health Council consists of national organizations, "including voluntary and governmental health agencies, professional and other membership associations, as well as civic organizations and business groups that have strong health interests. The three principal functions of the council are to help members promote the solution of national health problems of concern to the public, and to further improve governmental and voluntary health services for the public—at the state and local levels."

The problem now facing the committee was that the National Health Council, the fiscal agent for the committee and sponsor of the National Health Forum, had already mailed advanced publicity which read, "It is expected that preliminary reports of the President's Committee's history, methodology, findings, and tentative proposals will be available prior to the forum so that preregistered participants will have the opportunity to study this material in advance."

The brochure went on to explain that forum participants would have an opportunity to probe the data compiled by the committee and to examine its proposals. However, the full committee had not yet examined the draft of the report proposed by the staff. A lengthy, heated discussion on the report followed. More problems were likely to appear at the forum meeting in New Orleans, which was only two weeks away.

The premature decision by McNerney, also president-elect of the National Health Council, and Richard P. McGrail, president of the council and ex officio member of the President's Committee, created many conflicts within the entire committee.

At this stage of my growing dissent, it was obvious that the boys had a plan—long before many of us had a chance to provide input. The President's Committee report was becoming more bogus by the day. It was a matter of not accepting the committee's findings that highly prioritized the role of health education in bringing healthier lives to our people. The leadership of the committee directed emphasis toward the commercial world, which relied on highly competitive advertising of prescription medicines, health education limited to medical care providers, less control of false claims in both treatment and prevention, and promoting related legislation to benefit the powers that be in the health-care industry. This circumstance was such a personal and professional disappointment at a time in history when we had valid information on preventing disease and improving health by merely educating the young and the rest of us to establish and maintain our health through lifelong learning.

The subcommittee reports, including the School Health Report from the Subcommittee on Education, were received but not reviewed or acted upon by the committee. Materials presented to the committee included an additional position paper and a schematic for a National Center for Health Education, proposed by the staff. A national center included the concept of regional centers for health education and proposed locations for the centers. All were to be located in cities where regional hearings were held with the exception of one in Miami, the site of the 1972 Republican Convention. Emphasis was placed on political expediency rather than on the validity of the report content since the attempt was to create recommendations that could be used in Nixon's reelection campaign.

McNerney, who was on the Republican Platform Committee, made a motion that the work of the committee be extended beyond the May 31, 1972, deadline and that staff be authorized to seek funding for that extension at the rate of $15,000 per month.

> Mr. McNerney reported that because of the president's trip to Moscow, May 22, and the enormous volume of work that must be processed plus the intervention of the national political conventions, it was important that the initiatives and interest generated by the committee not be allowed to come to an abrupt halt with the formal submission of its report.

McNerney's motion was seconded and subsequently approved by the committee. Once again, the source of funds to support the work of the committee was undefined.

Siegfried wanted the committee to explore—with top HEW officials—the feasibility of assuming major responsibility for consumer health education. It was agreed that Weingarten would contact Secretary Richardson or Assistant Secretary Merlin DuVal, to whom President Nixon referred us during his earlier meeting with the committee.

THE PRESIDENT'S REPORT UNVEILED

On schedule, the printed report, "An Analysis of Testimony and Reports Given to the President's Committee on Health Education" by Melvin H. Rudov et al. (American Institute of Research) was presented to the committee. The forward of the report read:

> During the analysis of the testimony, a series of descriptions of programmatic activities were encountered. They ran the gamut of brief descriptions of activities to fairly comprehensive discussions of the objective methodologies and outcomes of specific large-scale programs. In almost all cases, discussions

of the products of these programs were insufficient for us to evaluate. We do not think that we can point to any specific program and say that it was effective, ineffective, or applicable to other communities. What we have done in this report is highlight the programs and provide whatever additional comments that seemed appropriate.

In the case of Los Angeles, more than fifty testimonies were given during the regional hearing; however, only seven were included in the Rudov report. *Why didn't the report include all the testimony? On what basis were selected presentations excluded?*

The absence of Simonds at the fourth full committee meeting—and his failure to notify me that the subcommittee meeting scheduled for the night before was canceled—seemed a bit unusual.

My workload for the committee, the coalition, and the university, including SEARCH, was mind-boggling. I was in excellent health and had been born with an abundance of energy—thanks to my heredity and my rearing. I valued hard work as a privilege, especially when I could see positive results. I could easily accomplish four man-years of work in one.

NATIONAL HEALTH FORUM MEETS

MARCH 20–22, 1972

The 1972 National Health Forum, sponsored by the National Health Council, was held in New Orleans. The topic was "People Keeping Healthy—Goals and Approaches to Consumer Health Education." The forum brought together 454 representatives of member agencies of the National Health Council, the President's Committee on Health Education, regional hearing participants, and others.

At the time of the forum, the Neenah 8 formally emerged after a yearlong feasibility study as the Coalition of National Health Education Organizations. The chief elected officers of all member organizations had signed a working agreement for a two-year period, 1972–1974. I served as the group's first coordinator from 1971 to 1974.

Emily Hammond, a delegate from the American Public Health Association, School Health Section, sent invitations to those health educators invited to the forum. As a result, approximately seventy participants met on Monday night to discuss their mutual interests and priorities in health education. Carlyon chaired the meeting. Each of the eight coalition representatives described the priorities for health education as defined by their respective organizations. With one exception, these priorities were defined in position papers prepared for the President's Committee. In keeping with plans that emerged from the third coalition mini conference in Ann Arbor, support was being generated for the coalition's unified position paper to the President's Committee on Health Education. According to the notes taken by delegates Hammond and Skiff, the meeting closed with an agreement to meet again the next night.

On Tuesday morning, the opening general session of the forum began with greetings from Larry and McNerney, now wearing three hats—vice chair for the President's Committee, president of the Blue Cross Association, and president of the National Health Council. The "Sight and Sound" presentation, admittedly developed in a few days, was shown. Those assembled at the opening session were told the presentation was prepared primarily for President Nixon as it could dramatize the health-education needs of the nation more effectively than the written report, a puzzling statement since the report had not yet been written, or had it?

Following the presentation, forum participants were asked to go to assigned discussion groups where they were to focus on selected questions from the discussion guide for the 1972 National Health Forum. I served as one of the group leaders. The participants wanted to comment on the presentation rather than the discussion guide. In general, comments about the presentation were negative. Several individuals said, "I don't believe the film is an appropriate method of reporting to the president." Also, members of the group did not like being told which questions in the guide they were to discuss.

Based upon preforum publicity, the expectations of those attending the forum were not being met. According to *Medical World News*, April 14, 1972:

> The participants had been told the "preliminary reports of the President's Committee findings and tentative proposals" would be made available. (When in fact, no such findings or proposals existed.) The participants were told that they would be able to "probe the data compiled by the committee." (No data were made available.) By lunch, some participants were seething. Comments such as "an insult to our intelligence" and "we're being used" were common reactions ... The luncheon speakers helped to sedate some delegates effectively ... and afterwards the meeting broke up into small groups. This gave further cause for resentment: Participants were arbitrarily assigned to groups to consider assigned questions." Also, they were asked to complete a structured "Attendee Response Sheet." Many claimed they were "responding to a directed position or course of action and that a spontaneous or democratic form of input from them was being thwarted."

Others were quoted as saying that they were pushed toward endorsing a national center, when such a center was inappropriate.

At the late afternoon reception honoring the President's Committee on Health Education, widespread discontentment was expressed by forum participants. The climate of the meeting was hostile; after a few drinks, the participants became less inhibited.

According to Hammond's and Skiff's minutes:

> On Tuesday night, approximately fifty health educators gathered again, and a number of them were very much concerned about procedures being employed

in the forum, questioned motives of the President's Committee and objected to being "used." Walter McNerney was invited to the session. He gave careful consideration to the feelings expressed, indicated that other groups were similarly concerned, and announced that the forum leadership had decided to dispense with the scheduled group meetings and to open discussion from the floor at the Wednesday meeting. He encouraged the coalition to have a spokesman to present our points of view and indicated that input from our group and organizations was welcomed both at the forum and after. Accordingly, representatives of the coalition agreed to present a coalition statement at the Wednesday session.

On Wednesday morning at eight o'clock, representatives of each of the organizations in the coalition met and agreed on the content of a coalition statement to be made by Carlyon. Rumors had reached me that I had been removed as coordinator of the coalition. This was to be expected since Carlyon was already serving as the coalition spokesperson at the forum. However, it was not true.

The second general session began at nine, and McNerney masterfully moderated the meeting. The forum's printed program copy was cast aside. All who wanted to speak out were given an opportunity to do so—consumer and provider groups alike. Among the consumer groups was the unified "RAZA" group representing those from a Spanish ethnic background.

Later, the RAZA group formulated their forum presentation by developing a position statement on "Health Education Needs and Concerns of Spanish Surnames, and Spanish-Speaking Americans," which was submitted to the President's Committee. From the position statement:

> Despite this administration's commitment to ensure meaningful participation and involvement from the

major ethnic and racial minorities, we collectively feel that the Spanish population, the second largest minority group in the nation has been excluded from participation in the work of the President's Committee on Health Education was established without a single representative of the nation's Spanish-surnamed population.

When Carlyon presented the coalition's position paper, it marked the first time in the history of our nation that professional health educators had spoken out as a national unified voice.

In their minutes, Hammond and Skiff wrote, "Mr. McNerney recognized the coalition explicitly and again expressed the committee's interest in receiving input from the coalition and indicated the committee looked forward with us in preparation of the president's report and requested that we send in a written statement to the committee."

Carlyon agreed to prepare such a draft for consideration by the other members.

On April 14, 1972, *Medical World News* reported that Carol D'Onofrio, delegate to the coalition from the Society of Public Health Education, Inc., and president of the society, said:

The forum had been a "source of frustration," since the input of the hearings was not available. And in the forum groups, she said, "We were structured into something that had been predetermined so that we did not have a voice in deciding what the major issues are; rather we were asked to respond to what someone else had decided." She likened the participants in the forum to a community of consumers and the President's Committee and its staff to providers. "This is what always happens," she said. "Our reaction is discontent, the suspicion that we are being used … Mr. McNerney handled it all with grace, sympathy, humor, and every evidence of sincerity. He explained where he could, apologized when a plan goof had been made, instantly accepted suggestions when feasible, promised full consideration in other cases, lowered temperatures and raised spirits ... He ended by announcing that the President's Committee would no longer try to meet the June deadline for its report. It would instead spend at least a couple of months more absorbing and taking into account what had been learned at the forum. "We have to do that," he said afterwards. "No health-education program can possibly be made to work without the support of these people."

Having witnessed a "turning of the tables" in the forum program, I was pleased at the end of the forum with the coalition's contribution and McNerney's promises. In *SOPHE News and Views,* D'Onofrio said, "The caucus on Tuesday night was instrumental in assuring that our views were positively and constructively presented on the second day."

Following the forum, a fifth meeting of the President's Committee was held while members were together. Most of the time was devoted to giving each member an opportunity to share reactions to the forum.

The minutes from the March 22 meeting read:

There was general discussion with Dr. Robert Laur as to what kind of information the committee was seeking from HEW. It was agreed that Laur was to obtain as comprehensive a picture as possible of HEW's role in health-education affairs.

Laur was a member of the staff council to the President's Committee on Health Education from HEW.

As the meeting culminated, attention turned to the report to the president. M. Alfred Haynes was a member of the committee and chairman of the Department of Community Medicine and associate dean of the Charles R. Drew Postgraduate Medical School.

Unless the proposed report more nearly conformed with what he believed the committee wanted, he would have to reconsider his involvement with the committee. He suggested that the time had now come for staff to draft a report which the committee could then use as a basis for its discussion. He said, "We need a consensus about what we mean by 'health education.'"

I was opposed to having the staff hand us a proposal for a report to the president without the committee first having discussed the development of such a report—and without a careful and complete analysis of the data that had been collected by the committee. Some subcommittee reports had not even been presented to the committee, including the report on school health, the most vital need for health education in America. Furthermore, I became frustrated when I realized the committee had been in operation for seven months and had not yet agreed on a definition of "health education."

As for the committee's frame of reference, the nature and meaning of health education remained unresolved, apparently by design. On February 18, 1971, President Nixon said:

> A series of new area Health Education Centers should also be established in places which are medically underserved—as the Carnegie Commission on Higher Education has recommended. These centers would be satellites of existing medical and other health science schools; typically, they could be built around a community hospital, a clinic, or HMO (Health Maintenance Organizations), which is already in existence. Each would provide a valuable teaching center for new health professionals, a focal point for the continuing education of experienced personnel, and a base for providing sophisticated medical

services, which would not otherwise be available in
these areas.

Unfortunately, for the future role of the health-education
profession, Nixon had misrepresented the term "health education"
and created a national wave of confusion. Our committee was now
feeling the frustration. If only President Nixon had referred to
health education as a learning process to favorably affect the health
of individuals and not misrepresent it with manpower training
programs that focused on preparing care providers to treat patients
instead of educating them.

The terms *health education* and *health educators* were being
misused and abused. Our national committee was doing little to
rectify these serious conflicts.

As the committee meeting ended, it was concluded that the next
meeting of the Committee on April 18 would be devoted largely to a
discussion of concepts as well as possible directions the committee
might consider recommending to the president.

The Commonwealth Fund made a grant to the National Health
Council to support the Council's Twentieth Annual National Health
Forum. According to the 1972 annual report of the fund, the forum
"was the occasion for the first public preview and review of the report
of the President's Committee on Health Education." Of course, this
did not actually happen, since there was no final report.

Simonds had written all members of the Subcommittee on
Education on March 16; however, before this letter arrived, I had left
for the National Health Forum in New Orleans.

The report that Simonds was now circulating and that Pauline
Carlyon had prepared was not to be confused with the "Preliminary
Report of Findings and Recommendations" prepared by the
subcommittee. This separate, seventy-five-page report, "Background
Papers: Review of Current Literature, Documents, and Reports," was
called the Carlyon Report. It resembled an unacceptable thesis more
than a subcommittee report. Carlyon's attached letter to Simonds
read in part:

> The attached report contains a review of current literature, documents, and reports submitted to the President's Committee as testimony and a brief historical review of earlier attempts to focus national commitment on school health education … I hope this adequately fulfills our agreement and meets with your approval as a background document that will be useful in the work of the President's Committee.

Obviously, as a subcommittee member, I wondered what the agreement between Simonds and Carlyon was.

On the same day that Simonds had written his letter to the subcommittee members, I had also written Simonds—and I had included a critique of the subcommittee's preliminary report.

At the forum, Simonds made no effort to have a meeting of the subcommittee or to plan the next steps as suggested in his letter. So many promises were never kept.

At that point in the process of creating a final report, I was reminded daily how difficult it was to make any progress on the meaning of "health education." Nearly every direction I took ended up on another pathway to my dissent.

PART 3

PATHWAYS TO DISSENT

JULY 20, 1972

On June 16, 1972, Weingarten had stated in a letter to me that the four Comprehensive School Health Education recommendations I presented would be very helpful. On July 17, he wrote me another letter.

> I am having difficulty with a fair number of the recommendations you have submitted for inclusion in the report as they pertain to comprehensive school health education programs. Some of the recommendations call for new legislation and new appropriations of enormous magnitude and I am loath to make such global recommendations without having a much clearer understanding of the parameters. In addition, the committee as a whole has not really discussed those items, and I think the committee itself would be embarrassed if either the president or the press were to ask how much money was involved if your school health proposals were implemented. We would have to confess we did not know, and I think this would tend to discredit the effort. I would

like to ask you to review the recommendations you have submitted and discuss them with Scott, and that they be more pragmatic and less "pie in the sky." The reason for this is that our major objective is to have the president accept and agree to implement our major recommendation. The White House staff has frequently told us and we know from reading the newspapers that the president backs away from global recommendations, which he believes are neither practical nor attainable. If we can get a national center established, it would be in a much better position to push for the longer-term recommendations, and we would run less jeopardy, in my opinion, of having the entire report discarded.

What had happened in the short time between his two letters? I think my previous letter to Larry on the lack of committee process had angered both of the rascals.

Later, Weingarten called me from the East Coast.

"Hello, Joy."

"Yes."

"This is Vic. Heath has approved your request to share future drafts of the report to the president with coalition delegates."

"Great," I responded. "I know the delegates will be very pleased. Thank you!"

Our conversation began on this positive note but rapidly moved to his displeasure over my letter to Larry. I was right. During the next half hour, he attempted to defend himself on each of the eight points in my letter. He became so angry that his voice cracked repeatedly; however, he continued to talk faster and louder, allowing me no chance to respond.

In talking over him, I said, "Please, Vic, you're taking the letter personally. It was directed to Larry—not you."

He did not react to my response. As he continued to yell at me, I hung up on him.

How can he show such disrespect for other committee members?

JULY 24, 1972

Among my many concerns were the report of the Subcommittee on Education and the integration of this document into the final report of the total committee. At this point, the subcommittee and its work appeared destined for failure, which is why I requested another subcommittee meeting from Simonds. Simonds appeared to agree with the request, but he ultimately undermined the effort by demanding a quorum in attendance and additional funds to cover travel and lodging. With these requirements, it was unlikely such a meeting would ever occur. The process of reviewing and approving the final subcommittee report could easily be done by mail. The door was closed.

Along with a copy of the second draft of the final report, Weingarten's cover letter said, "At this stage of the committee's work, insofar as the White House is concerned, the president's major concern was for a recommendation on the desirability of a new entity. The administration has its own timetable as to when it would like to meet with the committee on its major recommendation." Since the committee had already made a commitment to a new national entity, the White House was not really interested in anything else.

D'Onofrio's remarks from the forum rang in my ears. She said, "The local people and their committees are being ignored." Initially she appeared out of step, but she later fell in line with her troops. As for any committee timetable, it was apparently to fluctuate with the whims of the administration. The initial charge of the committee was forgotten or ignored.

EARLY FINAL REPORT DRAFTS

On July 24, I received the second draft of the report. I had the task of writing another critique.

Weingarten claimed that my first critique arrived too late. *Sorry about that; the second critique will be before the deadline.* I did a fourteen-hour marathon review of the second draft. I carefully completed a ten-page evaluation; it was done systematically and specifically focused on the president's charge to the committee. Even though Carlyon was to have sent delegates of the National Health Forum copies of the draft report prior to sending it to the president, perhaps there was still some hope that we could ensure the future of the health-education profession.

It was my first comprehensive and microscopic review of the president's report. I read and reread the second draft of the report. My critique of the report required ten pages of responses to errors, omissions, and misconceptions within the report. A new section, "The Role of the Coalition of National Health Education Organizations" was also submitted to clarify the importance of including coalition representation on the board of the National Center for Health Education, which should be renamed the "President's Committee on Health Education Confusion."

> Beginning in May of 1972, a study to explore the feasibility of an alliance of all professional health-education organizations was initiated. Within a year, the first coalition of national health-education organizations was formed to mobilize the resources of the profession for the expansion and improvement of citizen health in the United States. The National Center for Health Education needs the support and services of the coalition for many valid reasons.
>
> For example, the coalition
>
> - provides a linkage to all professional health-education groups at national, regional, and local levels;
> - represents those health-education professionals who could offer creative and dynamic

leadership, who have full-time careers in the profession, who serve in diversified settings, who specialize in various aspects and components of health-education programs, and who have special competencies relating to educational and behavioral change;

- can ensure the relevance of the center's program to the needs of the people since it has direct access to networks of providers and consumers and is capable of quickly and efficiently mobilizing and polling these resources.

It is recommended that the coalition be represented on the board of directors of the National Center for Consumer Health Education, and that through the coalition's involvement on the board of directors and on the board committees, they participate in decision-making processes associated with the establishment of policy for the center. Eight of the twenty-seven members of the board of directors should be representatives from the coalition. It is recommended that the National Center for Consumer Health Education establish advisory committees to function on a continuing basis in relation to each of the five major "divisions" of the center. These committees would monitor planning, implementation, and evaluation operations associated with the work of each "division." Further, that professional health educators recommended by the coalition serve on each of these "division" committees.

JULY 31, 1972

I received a memorandum from Weingarten announcing the August 17 meeting of the full committee to be held at the J. Walter Thompson Company in New York. With no agenda, the purpose of the meeting was to review the draft of the report to the president.

"This will probably be the last full meeting of the committee prior to our meeting with the president," concluded Weingarten.

AUGUST 2, 1972

Because of the letters I had sent in July, I now had a backlog of correspondence. I disappointingly observed Weingarten using a scare tactic to deter dissents from committee members. No one wanted to write a dissent that would be counter-dissented with no opportunity to respond. That would be a violation of due process.

This act by Weingarten certainly initiated my consideration of dissent—unless the issues that were still pending could be resolved.

AUGUST 4, 1972

In a letter, Weingarten made a major effort to respond to several points in my second draft critique. Three key items emerged from his letter: the coalition's role, position papers, and minority reports.

THE COALITION'S ROLE

"Your suggestion," stated Weingarten, "that the coalition be represented on the board of directors of the proposed center ... I would recommend against it because we are not recommending any specific organization be officially represented on the board."

He spoke of the coalition as one organization. It was not. It was a combination of eight organizations, all of which had the common mission of health education. The center needed this representation and balance of professional health educators.

He said, "I know that you are pushing for a major role for the coalition, but I believe that belongs in another arena—not this one—and I hope that upon reflection, you will agree."

I replied, "This indeed is the health-education arena—and others may belong elsewhere."

POSITION PAPERS

In my second critique of the report, I asked, "Who was commissioned to write position papers? Who made the decision to commission selected individuals to write those papers? Do we have a collection of commissioned position papers?"

Weingarten replied, "I commissioned position papers based upon recommendations and suggestions from various staff and committee members ... Some of the major papers have been described and have been distributed to all committee members several times."

According to the minutes of the President's Committee Meeting, dated February 10, 1972, the position papers had been commissioned by the committee.

My remaining questions regarding the position papers were never answered.

MINORITY REPORTS (DISSENTS)

Although I had indicated in my critique that all committee members should have a fair and equal opportunity to submit minority reports if we couldn't resolve issues, I was informed that "dissents will be published along with counter-dissents!" Unfortunately, the dissenter cannot react to the counter-dissenter's written response published in the report.

This was just the beginning of many threats made over the months ahead. Fortunately, I was not alone. The number of other members sharing my dissatisfaction was increasing, ultimately resulting in half of the committee.

FINAL REPORT CHALLENGES

AUGUST 8, 1972

Several communiqués presented issues that persisted throughout the final report drafting process. Many paths that one could easily take in making a dissent on the final report to the president were identified by Joseph Beirne in a letter to me:

> I have to agree with you that the apparent intention of the committee to "think small" is the wrong approach. In my May 24 "Individual Views," I explained why I had to abstain from voting at the May 15 meeting. I do not believe the committee and the National Center for Consumer Health Education can succeed unless each holds to a recommendation for significantly large amounts of money and commitment. I hope the rest of the committee will give great consideration to your view, which I value having.

After draft five, the additional drafts were never numbered—and it became difficult for one to know which draft they had or if it was the same draft that other individuals were talking about. The first four drafts were by committee members. The fifth draft was written by Syd Harris, a well-known columnist who was given $5,000 to prepare the draft. This draft was also not approved by the committee. I wrote the sixth draft, which was never approved or disapproved by the committee. The seventh draft presumably was written by Eddie Miller of Blue Cross. The eighth draft was written by the director, and apparently was a compilation of earlier drafts, including portions of the Miller draft and my drafts.

The general feeling at the last subcommittee meeting was to have another meeting or at least a conference call, but nothing ever happened. Therefore, after the fifth draft, there was never another meeting of the full committee. Decisions were made by a few individuals, and events were closed to those of us not in the "in group."

During these latter efforts in drafting the final report, one member of the committee in "Big Business" failed to communicate directly with the other committee members. Instead, his staff communicated and interpreted for him. Often, his staff members presented his bias, including derogatory statements about other committee members.

The committee never acted on drafts six, seven, or eight, but we were finally asked to vote on draft nine.

In addition to the loss of our efforts at drafting, materials from regional hearings, general correspondence, and information from the National Health Forum were ignored.

AUGUST 17, 1972

The process of assembling the final report was pitiful. Portions of proposed content were always missing. The minutes of the committee meeting presented some of the issues that were never resolved and resulted in growing dissatisfaction among many members.

In an attempt to clarify the position of the health educator, I wrote "The Role of the Health-Education Profession."

THE ROLE OF THE HEALTH-EDUCATION PROFESSION

Across the nation, consumers are successfully being involved in policy-making processes associated with the delivery of health and educational services. Ethnic minorities and women are beginning to receive equal opportunities in the employment field. However, unprecedented inequalities still remain unsolved within the professional family. For example, flagrant inequalities exist between health educators and other members of the health professions. This situation must be remedied before health educators can make a major contribution to the health of our nation.

Too often, physical educators dominate the destiny of health educators in schools, and physicians dominate the fate of health educators in health-care settings. It must be recognized that, while physicians and physical educators may be supportive of health-education programs and may personally assume some health-education responsibilities, they are not professionally trained health educators. For example, physicians may be licensed to perform surgery in operating rooms, but they are not certified to teach health education in public school classrooms.

Professionally trained health educators must have an optimum opportunity to participate in policy-making and program-planning functions associated with their profession at all levels. This is particularly true with reference to their role in the newly proposed National Center for Consumer Health Education. The latest report to the president does not reflect the leadership role that the health-education profession rightfully deserves and is capable of assuming. The opportunity to remove the prejudicial barrier that stands between their professional capability and achievement is lost. The Coalition of National Health Education Organizations, which represents all professional associations in the health-education programs, must not be alienated. Health educators, belonging to member organizations of the coalition, are the vital links between health-education consumers and providers. Their decision-making powers must be recognized and utilized in the center. To do otherwise would be hypocrisy, and only the American people stand to lose.

SEPTEMBER 5, 1972

Given my inability to integrate several critical segments related to the future of health education into the final report, I scheduled a dinner with Clarence J. Brown Jr. to alert him about upcoming legislation related to the President's Committee on Health Education. The critical items discussed over dinner included potential legislation for school health education and representation from the coalition on the new national center.

ADDITIONAL PATHWAYS

The following excerpts were taken from several hundred pages of original documentation of the committee process. These represent examples of corruption and related threats that took place throughout the process of assembling the final report.

SEPTEMBER 20, 1972

Upon returning from the full committee meeting in Chicago, a letter from Simonds was waiting for me. First of all, it confirmed that there would be no school health monograph due to budget restrictions and no subsequent subcommittee meetings since Simonds decided that a minimum of three members must be present. We had not met since Mother's Day, and we would not meet again—even though the work of the committee was incomplete.

SEPTEMBER 29, 1972

I received a copy of a letter Simonds had written to Weingarten stating that his schedule would not permit him to attend the editorial subcommittee meeting scheduled for October 3. "I hope Joy Cauffman can attend as we discussed."

Like any integrating process, there are always conflicts and pains. It has taken considerable time to come up with a blend of the first five drafts, including suggestions from the past full committee meeting. My secretary notified McNerney's office that I would be at the subcommittee meeting.

I was obviously being considered by the decision makers for an attempt to gain my support of the final report. The assumption must have been that I would vote for its approval if I had a major role in actually writing the report.

OCTOBER 1–3, 1972

I completed my write-up of the national center prior to leaving for the editorial subcommittee meeting in Chicago. The meeting was attended by McNerney, Joseph T. Painter, A. C. Nielsen Jr., Weingarten, and me. Painter was with the Ledbetter Clinic Association and a member of the board of directors for Blue Cross/Blue Shield of Texas. Nielsen was the president of the A. C. Nielsen Company, the world's largest in marketing.

During the initial socializing, Weingarten shared with McNerney a new paperback his wife had written, during which I learned that Weingarten was a consultant to the top brass of Blue Cross. There was no agenda for the meeting. It was informal but task-oriented.

I had completed the national center write-up and shared it with the committee members. As the meeting progressed, I was given more responsibility for rewriting the full report in a manner similar to the national center section. Weingarten agreed to send me his personal notes from the last full committee meeting and this subcommittee meeting since no official minutes were being taken.

McNerney indicated that he would call me at my hotel before he went to dinner.

Painter and I walked back to our hotel. It was a great break after such a long session. Painter said, "I will have the report reviewed by the AMA."

I didn't respond directly to his remark, but I was surprised that the AMA had access to the report and influenced its content, but the Coalition of Health Educators had no contact.

Shortly after I reached my hotel room, the phone rang.

McNerney said, "Joy, my family and I have a dinner party tonight with Nielsen, but I would like to see you for a few minutes."

"Okay, I will be here."

When McNerney arrived, he was in a rush and came directly to the point. "You are going to rewrite the report?"

"Yes. I said I would."

"You will meet the deadline?"

"I will do my best."

Although he appeared overly concerned about my commitment, he said, "Joy, I know you can do it. You will have to be one of the committee members who has a picture taken with the president."

I smiled as he went off to his dinner party. When I reflected on this interaction, I believed McNerney thought I would vote for it if I wrote the report. I never said I wouldn't vote for the report. In fact, I strongly wanted to vote for the report—as long as it was a sound blueprint for future action.

OCTOBER 4–8, 1972

I spent my early mornings and evenings working on rewriting the report. I talked to my chairman, Harold Mazur, at USC. "I will be working late each evening on the report to the president during the next several weeks."

He said, "I'm pleased you are making a major contribution to the report. Be sure you are paid well for your services."

"I'm accepting no money for my work. It is my responsibility as a committee member."

I didn't appreciate working alone at night since my office was in an area that had been plagued by burglaries. On one particular night, when I was working past midnight, several typewriters were stolen from our floor. While talking with the police, I realized I had passed one of the robbers on my way to the restroom that evening. I really didn't need additional fears for my safety.

Integrating material from previous reports became particularly difficult. I was struck by the fact that—in spite of new information—little had changed from the previous drafts. It was almost as if a small group of individuals from the Rockefeller Committee was trying to hold the line to predetermine the content. I was amazed that new evidence sanctioned by the committee was not included in the drafts. I guess that was why the controlling leaders always requested the drafts for their editing prior to dissemination to the remaining committee members.

OCTOBER 9, 1972

I received a letter from A. C. Nielsen Jr. informing me that his son was starting a medical internship at Los Angeles County Hospital. Also, he acknowledged my contributions at the subcommittee meeting. His friendship—along with his comrades—appeared to have the hidden intent of preventing my dissent.

OCTOBER 27, 1972

I worked nearly around the clock to complete the sixth draft. I had completed a comprehensive content analysis of the total report, had eliminated duplications, reorganized existing data into meaningful categories and subcategories, and—when necessary and consistent with committee wishes—filled in gaps to provide continuity to the report.

I called McNerney. "The sixth report is on its way. Considering the limitations under which I was working, I believe it is a good report—one that the committee will support. The report is being sent to you, Larry, the other members of the editorial committee, and Weingarten."

McNerney said, "Only send a copy to me and Weingarten."

I was so exhausted that I didn't even ask why. "Okay. I'm on my way to the airport."

"Wait a minute. I plan to be in Los Angeles next week for a celebration on behalf of the new Blue Cross president of Southern California. Will you join me for the banquet and dance at the Century Plaza Hotel?"

"I will know on Monday."

"Good, I will talk to you then."

When I returned to my office in the morning, the other addressed report envelopes were missing from my desk. They had been sent by my dedicated secretary!

DRAFT SIX

As I look back, I am glad I had prepared the sixth draft of the report. It represented a composite critique of all the earlier drafts. In addition, it provided tangible evidence when compared with the ninth draft with which certain corporate giants in the nation had castrated the health-education leadership.

OCTOBER 30, 1972

McNerney called me at home on Monday. My husband answered the phone.

"Is Dr. Cauffman there?"

"No, she is at work."

Being the politician he is, McNerney said, "I want you to know that your wife's work in rewriting the report was outstanding."

My husband said, "I know Joy will be pleased with your comments. She has worked long hours, but she has the patience and ability to handle assignments of this type."

When I reached home, I called McNerney. "I apologize for not calling you earlier in the day. I'm unable to accept your invitation to the banquet and dance. Perhaps I can take a rain check for some future event in the Los Angeles area."

It probably would have been a very challenging evening.

After a long pause, he said, "Sure."

"Have fun. I will be in touch after the report arrives."

DRAFT SEVEN

NOVEMBER 4–5, 1972

When the seventh draft of the report arrived from Weingarten, the first fifty-five pages had been written by someone else, probably Eddy Miller of Blue Cross. Parts of the work I had done, now identified as the sixth draft of the report, were haphazardly attached to the end of the seventh draft. The strokes of the editor's pen had been devastating to the content, which had not been retyped, only merely cut and sloppily patched together. Since the additions were in a different font, they stood out boldly.

I had been asked by the committee and the members of the editorial subcommittee to rewrite the report. Did they assume it would be easier to flush down the toilet if I wrote my perspective of the report? I felt as if I had been used as a joke—I wished I could have been a fly on the wall.

When I shared this with Congressman Brown, he said, "That's great, Joy, but for God's sake, do not take any money."

I think Harold Mazur's warning had contained an ulterior motive.

I said, "I have not—and would never—considered taking money. You know me better than that."

"Yes, I really do. Sorry for my hasty comment."

When the work was completed, there was an initial attempt to cover up my efforts as if they had never existed. In addition, there was a latent attempt to butcher my hard work. In the absence of official minutes from the last full committee and editorial subcommittee meetings, there were still a few scattered pieces of evidence that revealed the true nature of this tragedy.

I wrote Weingarten, with copies to those who attended the last editorial subcommittee meeting, stating my dismay over the contents of the most recent draft—and for the first time I stated my decision to dissent from the President's Committee's final report unless there was reconsideration of its structure and content.

The next day, I wrote a similar letter to the other members of the President's Committee.

NOVEMBER 11, 1972

Simonds and Shapiro were reporting on the activities of the President's Committee at the general session of the Society of Public Health Education (SOPHE), in Atlantic City.

When I walked into the room, Weingarten saw me and appeared aghast.

Shapiro abruptly came down from the stage and kissed and hugged me—just for the audience. Since I had not been invited to be on the panel and was not expected to be present, Simonds and Shapiro appeared nervous about what I might say.

I was not asked to speak.

At the close of the session, many people gathered around me as I moved through the crowd.

"Why weren't you on the panel?" they asked.

"I wasn't asked."

They uttered expressions of foul play.

The retaliation toward a dissent that I had not even written yet had started.

THREATS OF RETALIATION

NOVEMBER 12, 1972

I was also in Atlantic City to make a presentation before the Conference of State and Territorial Directors of Public Health Education. As I entered the conference room, someone handed me a copy of the program. I noticed that Weingarten was also on the program as the luncheon speaker. I was the second speaker of the day and was to speak immediately after the midmorning break.

After the break, I was asked to sit at the head of the table. I looked up and noticed that Weingarten had just arrived. He apparently had come early to hear what I had to say. He spotted me and walked over to where I was seated at the head table.

He stated that he was very angry because I had dissented from the report. He demonstrated his anger by swearing intermittently, claiming he would get even by seeing that

- my professional and personal credibility were destroyed;
- I would have no further opportunity for involvement in national health-education affairs;
- I would not receive my promotion at USC; in fact, I would lose my tenured position;

- I would lose my current research grant, SEARCH, and receive no further grants from the government.

Weingarten's outburst was unexpected, particularly in this setting. I was in no position to respond to his threats—or to leave the meeting. I rearranged my chair to avoid seeing Weingarten. I tried to remain calm. I made my presentation about the work of the Coalition of National Health Education Organizations, responded to questions, and remained for lunch as planned. Due to another speaking engagement that evening, I left the luncheon before Weingarten spoke about the work of the President's Committee on Health Education.

I will never forget the impact of this incident on my commitment to dissent. I called two of my close friends about what had happened. They both knew Weingarten and indicated that nothing he said or did would surprise them. They agreed that no response was best for that kind of behavior.

Many questions came to mind. Would these threats be carried out? Who could assist him? Had Joe Bierne, another dissenter, received such threats? Once again, in this unbelievable circumstance, time would tell.

NOVEMBER 15, 1972

A few days after the APHA general session, I ran into Weingarten again in a corridor. There was no way to avoid a face-to-face encounter. From a distance, he began to wave his arm and point at me. He said, "Goddamn you. I will see that your career is destroyed. No promotion, no national limelight, and no research support for you. To prevent you from hurting me further, I was responsible for excluding you from presenting at this general session. There was no picture of you in the program. This is only the beginning."

I had never anticipated this kind of behavior from colleagues who were selected to represent the people. I believe my dissent was not totally due to the politically driven outcomes of the committee process—it was also to maintain the rights of dissent as a vital part of our freedom and future.

WHY SUCH THREATS AND RETALIATIONS?

In considering the cause of such threats and retaliations, I am certain my dissent became the main cause of efforts to destroy my life. Victor Weingarten became a vicious spider with large webs throughout the country. He led the effort to retaliate against me in keeping with this repeated and witnessed threats. Why such retaliation for dissenting as a member of a committee?

Weingarten had difficulty accepting my recommendations, which often challenged his position as director of the President's Committee. It threatened his image and role with the other members of the committee. He claimed I had a personal plan—while his plan manipulated the entire committee process to support predetermined outcomes.

My ongoing efforts to change the process culminated in personal threats from Weingarten, due primarily to his anger at having to cope with me and several other members of the committee who shared many of my concerns. I was one of many who initiated reactions threatening Weingarten beyond his level of tolerance. His similar anger and threats continued.

I believe Weingarten found it difficult to accept my concerns and criticisms as a woman.

Another likely cause of retaliation was my challenging his predetermined recommendations that were designed to support new legislation that gave continued control of health care to the key players—health insurance providers, pharmaceutical companies, and certain health-care provider groups. I believe his accusations were projections of his own intents. Nevertheless, health educators were ignored in addition to the people who should have had opportunities to improve their health and reduce costs through health education.

The financial affairs of the committee presented another issue that was totally isolated within the leadership. At the beginning, committee members were given some financial information. After the first few months, additional financial reports were never provided. The aggressive nature of personal threats and damage to Ron Linder's car were perhaps the result of fear among the leadership that we might initiate an investigation of the committee's possible use of funds for the Watergate and Ellsberg break-ins—in addition to our relentless documentation of committee activities with the intent to share it with the public. The release of our book with the detail provided herein at the time could have been another contribution to Nixon's impeachment. We may never know, but the committee's financial activities might have been the most serious threat to Weingarten and his team at the time of my dissent.

The threats and retaliations had the intent of getting me to give up and leave my professional life behind.

After twenty-five years of stress and two strokes, I feel the door is finally closed. I am thankful to have the opportunity to share this part of my story with you.

The mission has expanded from preserving the future of health education to also preserving the right to dissent. Now, I must move forward and write my dissent.

PART 4
THE DISSENT(S)

NOVEMBER 20, 1972

On Monday, I was back in Los Angeles. McNerney's memorandum from November 8 with the eighth draft of the report was waiting for me.

"Please read it as soon as practicable and send your comments to me. I will set November 16 as the deadline ... At this point, a date with the president can be made."

Since my response to the draft was due four days earlier, I responded:

> I feel only dismay at this point in time to be faced
> with content, so unresponsive to the stated purpose,
> and so devoid of quality ... It would take several days
> of concentration to identify and translate into writing
> the errors, distortions, omissions, and overlaps.

JOINT DISSENTS

NOVEMBER 22, 1972

Haynes and I had talked several times about combining our dissents for the final report. We thought more impact would be made if both of us agreed to the same issues and recommendations.

In the evening after work, Haynes came to my home. He met my husband and son, and we socialized a little. Haynes and I worked into the wee hours of the morning preparing our joint dissent.

After a few refreshments, he said, "I am going to Catalina Island this weekend, but I will be home on Sunday evening. Can you have our dissent draft typed? If it is not too inconvenient, just place a copy in my mailbox. Then I can review it before we meet again on Monday evening."

NOVEMBER 23–27, 1972

Over the weekend, I prepared the draft of our joint dissent, but I was unable to deliver it to his home by Sunday evening. On Monday morning, when I reached my office, I had a letter from McNerney. It was a follow-up to his earlier telegram.

I noted deceptive tactics in McNerney's letter. I had never been an official member of the editorial subcommittee. I only substituted for Simonds at the one meeting. Now it was made to look as if I was an original member of the editorial subcommittee from the beginning. I assumed that—as an alleged member of the subcommittee—they thought I would not dissent. That way, the others would approve the final report, since many committee members agreed with me on several issues.

When I reached home that evening, Haynes's wife called to report that he was delayed and would call me immediately upon arriving home. I spent several hours waiting for his call.

Finally, he called. "I'm sorry I was delayed. I won't be able to write the dissent with you. I have talked with Howard and Vic. Vic says you have sent letters to Secretary Richardson."

"That is true, but you also sent letters to Richardson. What is the issue?" I reminded him that Secretary Richardson was an ex officio member of the committee.

Haynes didn't clarify the issue. Our conversation was short and uninformative.

As I hung up, I was convinced that several people had gotten to Haynes—and his position was somehow being compromised. I wondered why he had changed his vote. Was he being rewarded or threatened? In putting three communiqués together, it appeared obvious that Haynes had made a quick and radical change in his view of the committee and the nature of his response due to the possible price of his dissent.

On November 20, Haynes wrote a letter to the committee members.

> I must honestly tell you that I am ashamed of the final document, which will no doubt prove to be a monument of mediocrity. I am not proud of being a member of a president's committee … I regret that we have missed a unique opportunity to make a really significant contribution to the cause of consumer health education.

On November 28, Ella Strother responded, "I believe that you and Dr. Cauffman understood and have portrayed my position. Therefore, I would like to be included in the minority report that you intend to submit to the President's Committee."

Two days later, Weingarten sent a statement to all committee members:

> Dr. Alfred Haynes has asked me to write to you to say that a letter he sent commenting on the draft of the proposed report to the president was based on an earlier version and was not based on the draft currently being considered.

I later discovered through a fellow staff member of Haynes that "he received money for changing his dissent. Although he was to receive a certain amount of money, part of the total was taken away from him later."

What was his actual price for not dissenting?

Later, Haynes returned to play a major role in my life by arranging an international opportunity to lecture and consult in South Africa, enabling me to continue my contribution to the field of health education among professionals, patients, students, and the public. He became a special mentor at the crossroads of my life and contributed to my redemption, along with many others.

NOVEMBER 28, 1972

My dissent contained ten major points, including the fact that committee goals were left unfulfilled and committee procedures were irregular. Of paramount significance was the fact that five major points in my dissent pertained to leadership.

Looking back, I had prepared the sixth draft of the report, and it had been shafted. I was glad I had prepared the earlier draft since it represented a composite critique of the first five drafts and provided a basis against which I could compare the ninth draft. The overwhelming difference in the sixth and ninth drafts came into focus as I compared the recommendations within the two documents on an item-by-item basis. The recommendations in the sixth draft, which involved representation from the health-education profession and designated leadership roles for professional health educators, had been removed. The profession had been ignored.

MY DISSENT

GOALS LEFT UNFULFILLED

A careful analysis of the published report clearly demonstrates that: On November 28, 1972, I prepared a first dissent. It was based on the report of the President's Committee on Health Education dated December 15, 1972 (ninth draft), which was distributed to the total committee by the chairman of the editorial subcommittee on November 22, 1972, for approval or dissent within ten days. Subsequently, the December 15, 1972, report was altered but without approval of the total committee. (This altered draft was dated December 11, 1972.)

On December 29, 1972, I prepared a second dissent, which is basically the same as my first dissent, but which takes into account alterations appearing in the tenth draft. This second dissent is based on the report of the President's Committee on Health Education dated December 11, 1972 (tenth draft), which was distributed at some later date to some members of the committee before it was submitted to the secretary of Health, Education and Welfare on December 14, 1972. (If the reader is confused by the dates given, please note that the report dated December 15, 1972, preceded the report dated December 11, 1972.)

The goals set forth in the president's charge to the committee and held forth to the general public were never fully achieved by the committee due to undue process.

COMMITTEE PROCEDURES IRREGULAR

The report represents the end product of over a year's work by the committee. Efforts leading to the report were conducted under conditions in which staff was permitted to usurp committee responsibility and in which committee leadership was ineffective in pursuing the president's assignment. Processes involved in producing the report have not contributed to its credibility. For example, information submitted to the staff often either never reached or was censored before reaching the full committee. Committee leadership involved its members in meaningless exercises and failed to properly use their talents and resources.

The achievement grade is F for failure. The procedures were irregular due primarily to the underlying politics within and surrounding the committee. With no regular procedures, the control of the outcomes was held by the leadership.

THE NATURE AND MEANING OF HEALTH EDUCATION DISTORTED

The substance of the report becomes distorted because of its failure to clearly focus on the subject of health education. Obviously, health education should be the central issue since both the title of the committee and the charge to the committee explicitly state this responsibility. However, the report improperly emphasizes ancillary issues, such as the history of medicine and public health, health problems, and health care. In the process of interweaving health education with other ancillary issues, essential distinctions are not always clearly delineated and viable linkages are not always provided between the ancillary issues and health education. Thus, the total conceptualization of the report lacks rational thinking, continuity, suitable perspective, and integration. Because of these significant deficiencies in the report, the nature and meaning of health education are heavily clouded, and the report becomes less than professional in its misdirected effort to interpret health education to the public.

Health is the total physical, mental, social, and spiritual well-being of the individual and not merely the absence of disease or infirmity. Health education consists of organized learning experiences with objectives and curriculum designed to maintain and improve the health of self and others. Health education within our schools is the essential foundation of basic facts and principles of good health, in addition to facilitating the interpretation of current information flooding the digital world today, much of which is false and profit motivated.

LEADERSHIP OPPORTUNITIES FOR PROFESSIONAL HEALTH EDUCATORS DENIED

The report does not provide the leadership opportunities that professional health educators rightfully deserve and are capable of assuming. The chance to remove any prejudicial barrier that stands between professional capability and achievement is lost. For example, the report should, but does not, specify that the National Center for Health Education will have both an administrator and a health-education director. The director should be a professional health educator with a background and experience in community and school health education and should hold a position in the center that is analogous to a position held by a physician who is a medical director in a hospital. Further, the report should, but does not, specify that professional community and school health educators should share leadership roles for health education at high policy-making and administrative levels within federal, state, and local government.

One of the difficulties observed during Dr. Linder's and my years of developing postgraduate medical education programs at UCLA and USC, respectfully, was the lack of training among physicians on how to teach with increasing needs for alternative learning applications within our digital world. Most college professors in the health sciences do not have any training on how to teach. Yet they usually view themselves as true health educators.

Faculty participating in postgraduate medical education programs often thanked us for assisting in the development of their presentations, particularly support media, often used subsequently in their additional teaching responsibilities. The traditional lecture approach is rapidly becoming obsolete. Consumer and public health education are predominantly information-based, although many nonprofit health-related groups cosponsor local education programs for the public. True health education is based on being able to make informed decisions by applying the principles of the health sciences, which is best accomplished through formal health-education programs in our schools, not just rainy-day opportunities.

SUPPORT FOR CRITICAL HEALTH-EDUCATOR MANPOWER SHORTAGES OMITTED

The report reflects the need for increased health-educator manpower in the United States, particularly in early childhood, school, and hospital settings. At the same time, the report fails to recommend support of training programs for professional health educators, and it conversely recommends support of training programs for nonprofessionals, such as paramedics and volunteers who are to perform health-education functions. Extending nonprofessional manpower in health education without proportionate expansions in already depleted professional health-educator ranks places an unrealistic burden on existing manpower. Therefore, the federal government should, as a manpower priority, extend its present training programs for community health educators to include school health educators. The more than one hundred institutions of higher education in the United States that prepare professional health educators—and that are capable of contributing a strong basic health science input—should conduct these training programs.

We can no longer "let George do it." There are not enough "Georges" to go around. Our future depends first and foremost on professionally trained educators particularly at a time when high-technology-based learning is our future. In trying to interpret the suppression of health education, it appears that committee leaders were trying to control the future of health education to enhance business profits through health information most consumers cannot interpret. The promotion of medications over television and the Internet requires health-educated consumers to enhance sound decision making toward better health.

THE UNIFIED VOICE FOR THE HEALTH-EDUCATION PROFESSION IGNORED

The report discriminates against the Coalition of National Health Education Organizations representing the unified voice of the health-education profession and consisting of all national health-education organizations in the United States with identifiable health-educator memberships and ongoing health-education programs. This is apparent since only a single reference is made to the coalition in the table of organization for the National Center for Health Education. This single reference clearly shows that the coalition would have no direct role in establishing center policy. In an effort that anticipates mounting a comprehensive nationwide health-education program, it is inconceivable that the primary full-time providers of health-education services in this country are virtually ignored. Thwarting the profession dissipates valuable trained resources contributing to the nation's health. As a result, the American people stand to lose.

The coalition, composed of nine national health-education organizations, did not qualify to support the political goals of the President's Committee leaders. To not include our outstanding health-education leadership at the national level was criminal.

VALUE OF MASS MEDIA NOT FULLY RECOGNIZED

While no health-education program can be fully and effectively implemented through only mass media, it would have been important for the report to clearly specify the dimensions of mass media's involvement since media have potential for both favorably and unfavorably influencing the quality of life for millions of Americans. The report does pay passing attention to the subject of mass media in relation to the National Center for Health Education, but it otherwise neglects to encourage sound linkages between health-education practitioners and mass media specialists within both large networks and local outlets.

Mass media has become a melting pot for health issues, information, and advertising. Many prime-time television shows are based in part or completely on health problems. The interest in health is obvious. The challenge before us is to educate our people to understand what they are being told and what the true implications are for their health.

NATIONAL CENTER FOR HEALTH EDUCATION UNACCOUNTABLE TO THE NATION

The report projects "the operating budget of the center for the first five years would be $12–15 million" and "the program budget would be somewhat higher." The budget projections, however, do not specify major categories of anticipated expenditures and do not relate expenditures to functions of the center. Therefore, the specification of functional priorities within the center has not been delineated within the report. In addition, the report fails to develop a plan of evaluation, including accountability for center functions. Such an omission is particularly difficult to understand in light of the numerous findings and recommendations on the subject of evaluation within the report, and in view of the role the center will play in evaluating the health-education efforts of others. If clearly described evaluation programs apply to all other health-education programs, the center should not be immune; to the contrary, the center must play an exemplary role. Furthermore, since the center is to serve the American public, it must be accountable to the people. To do otherwise is hypocrisy.

Without health educators, the Center for Health Education remains fictitious.

THE AMERICAN PEOPLE, VICTIMS OF FALSE PROMISES

All who wished to testify at the regional hearings held in major cities across the nation during January

1972 were given an opportunity to be heard. Many speakers waited endless hours to testify and were promised that their presentations would be given careful attention. It is a grievous fault that the full committee demonstrates its failure to utilize the full range of information received in selecting major ideas for the report.

Following the National Health Forum in New Orleans in March 1972, *Medical World News* reported that the committee did not keep its promise to participants by providing preliminary findings at the forum. This was true. Participants at the forum, however, were assured by committee leadership that their input would be carefully considered by the full committee. This was not done. Even more distressing is the fact that the body of the report does not even mention the National Health Forum.

The National Health Forum was not mentioned in this report—since several issues raised within the forum were not conducive to the political intent of the committee leaders. Once again, the practice was to ignore conflicts that did not contribute to the predetermined intent.

IMPLEMENTATION AND FOLLOW-UP DISREGARDED

The report includes more than thirty recommendations under the label of "National Activities in Support of Health Education." The fact is that many of the recommendations address themselves to responsibilities that should be carried out by—or in cooperation with—state and local leadership. In addition, supportive evidence to clarify the recommendations and to make the implementations readily feasible are missing from the report. As examples, the report recommends that model laws for school health-education programs be encouraged, but it fails to suggest content to be included in such laws. The report further recommends that the nation's hospitals provide health-education programs, but it fails to suggest the nature and scope of such programs. The report should contain guidelines for immediate action and follow-up of the report at community, state, and national levels, and it should provide a blueprint for future planning and actions associated with a comprehensive nationwide health-education effort.

WEINGARTEN'S COUNTER-DISSENT

Dr. Cauffman's prime concern seems to be that she would like to have a larger role assigned to the "Coalition of National Health Education Organizations," which she currently heads. Contrary to her complaints, the coalition is recognized as one of the major—but not the sole—professional organizations that can play a role in implementing the committee's primary recommendation. Another prime concern of Dr. Cauffman relates to her apparent belief that the report ought to be more forceful in attempting to support the injection of professional health educators into virtually every walk of life wherein health education is important. Most of the committee was unable to support the extent and scope of these recommendations, albeit recognizing the importance of professional health educators as the report does. It seems apparent that professional health educators have important work to do in inducing enlarged public support for their activities.

We regret the misunderstanding which has led to Dr. Cauffman's complaint about the sharing of data. Data collected from all sources were made available, not to all members of all subcommittees, but to the appropriate subcommittees on which members served. Dr. Cauffman, for example, received all papers and testimony relating to school health education, her primary study area. No member received copies of all two thousand papers, seventy-one hours of testimony, reports, etc., although all committee members received a summary of analysis of all testimony at all regional hearings, especially prepared for the committee by the American Institutes for Research.

In addition, a major portion of one committee meeting was devoted to an exchange of experiences and information about members' participation in the eight regional hearings. And finally, Dr. Cauffman would prefer that there be included more details with respect to a number of the recommendations of the report. Most of the committee believed that such details should be left to the implementing responsibility of the proposed center and to the myriad public and private organizations whose work impacts upon effective health education.

Earlier, McNerney had asked all committee members to either dissent from or vote for the report. Now, for the first time, I see a new category entitled "Supplementary Statements." Apparently, some committee members were told at a later date that they could prepare supplementary statements. This act of discrimination reflected more corrupt committee leadership. This last-minute option was obviously created to reduce the number of dissenters.

In response to Weingarten's comments on my dissent, which I was not allowed to react to within the final report, virtually half of the committee (ten) either "dissented" or provided a "supplementary statement," three of whom used the word dissent. I was not alone in my dissatisfaction with the report. Weingarten focused on me as an individual and not on the real issues related to the suppression of professional health educators. His comments were in bad taste, ludicrous, and preposterous. Since I was such an activist and influenced many others, my dissent created feedback by my biggest enemy, Weingarten, and he continued to punish me for many years for not joining his political pack.

This book would not have been possible if Victor Weingarten hadn't retaliated against me. At the present time in history when we are finally taking a serious look at health-care reform, perhaps my story will have some positive impact on the importance of health education in expanding the quality of life, preventing disease, and ultimately reducing the costs of health care. If this tragedy of my life has some positive influence on the role of health education in the future, the retaliations will have been worth it. Perhaps, this was supposed to happen.

I viewed those who prepared supplementary statements as the "fence-post-sitters." They were much like pumpkins after Halloween—only to be eventually struck down by lightning, rain, snow, or severe wind.

I was pleased that Joseph Beirne's dissent had weathered the storm. He spoke of one of the issues, "The American People, the Victims of False Promises," in my dissent. "This report, as presented for final ratification by members of the committee, also does an injustice to the nearly three hundred citizens and health professionals who testified at the eight public hearings, in my view."

Ten years from now, it will be interesting to see if Beirne's following prediction comes true:

> I strongly believe that the National Center for Health Education, if formed within the framework of this report, will not be effective. And thus, in the future, it will be doubly difficult to do a proper job, because

of a need to undo what has been improperly entered upon.

Nearly four decades later, Beirne's prediction still remains true.

DECEMBER 18, 1972

Before the bogus report was sent to Secretary Richardson, many events had taken place behind the curtain of Blue Cross. The air was contaminated with acts of so-called friendly persuasion, threats, political promises, and bribes. In addition to the incidents already cited, I was told that McNerney was negotiating a large advertising contract with Seymour of the J. Walter Thompson Company. Thus, the air was further clouded by concomitant financial deals involving big business.

As I examined the final report, although my dissent was unchanged, other parts of the report had been altered. Have you ever voted on something, such as minutes or a report, and upon examining the final document discovered that substantial alterations had been made in the interim? So it was for the report that was finally sent to the president.

Of the nineteen committee members, with the death of Wilson and including ex officio members, nine voted for the report, eight prepared supplementary statements and two dissented.

VOTED FOR THE REPORT (8)

Leroy E. Burney
R. Health Larry
John Alexander McMahon
Walter J. McNerney
A. C. Nielsen Jr.
Joseph T. Painter
Elliot Lee Richardson
Dan Seymour

SUBMITTED SUPPLEMENTARY STATEMENTS (8)

M. Alford Haynes
Richard P. McGrail
C. Wrede Petersmeyer
Irving S. Shapiro
Charles A. Siegfried
Scott K. Simonds
J. Henry Smith
Ella Louise Strother

DISSENTED FROM THE REPORT (2)

Joseph A. Beirne
Joy G. Cauffman

Most individuals who read the report recognized that Weingarten was defensive. He picked on me as a person and ignored the real issues at hand.

UNDUE PROCESS

The committee as a whole had a small part in shaping its destiny. The leadership and staff had predetermined committee activities and outcomes. The staff prepared a prescribed final report in the absence of true committee involvement. I had served as a consultant on two presidential committees without any resemblance to this one.

The following observations represent a brief final summary of the undue process contributing to my dissent, which is now indelible within the final report:

COMMITTEE

The process by which the committee was directed was unorthodox and unstructured. Both conventional parliamentary procedures and committee protocol were absent. Committee leaders took advantage of the opportunity to manipulate the process to fulfill personal and political goals. Several committee members were not really committed to the task at hand. They attended meetings sporadically or left early. Suggested agenda items were always held toward the end of the meetings, when the quorum was lost or the topic became delayed to the next meeting, and ultimately were dropped from future consideration.

EDITORIAL SUBCOMMITTEE

At the last meeting of the editorial subcommittee, there were plans for a follow-up meeting, but it was never held. There was also discussion of having a conference call; that also never took place. The die had been cast; there was no need for a meeting when there would be no change.

REGIONAL HEARINGS

Throughout the regional hearings, the health-education success stories and the leaders in the field—who often accomplished their goals at great personal sacrifice—were ignored. Nearly all input from the hearings was discarded or placed in storage.

THE CHARGE

Committee leadership promoted the concept of a national center at the expense of all other considerations. They justified their actions by claiming that the White House had established this priority. Why didn't the president's charge reflect it? Once the leadership obtained approval of the recommendation for a national center, other recommendations were routinely refuted or lost.

MINUTES

Verbal statements within the minutes, when provided, were written to suit the desires of those in power—the leadership of the committee.

STAFF

Staff members often misrepresented committee members and only took direct orders from the leadership. They often made derogatory statements to others that reflected the thoughts of their bosses. One McNerney staff member told my secretary in a negative manner that I was "vehement" on various issues and needed to relax.

CONTENTS OF THE REPORT

The fundamental principles of survey research were not followed in the committee's work. The report was totally written to support the political motives of those in charge—without accepting the true meaning of health education. To provide no guidelines for community involvement in health-education programs, after initiating community interest and participation, was misleading and tragic.

COMMITTEE FINANCES

The finances were kept private between committee leaders only. There was no official budget, and many rumors pointed toward funds that may have been placed outside the committee, including Watergate and related incidents. We may never know.

MAY 7, 1973

I sent a memorandum to coalition delegates regarding the status of the President's Committee report. My remarks were based on a recent letter from Weingarten. I took a stand with respect to not preparing a coalition position statement on the report until we had it in hand.

SEPTEMBER 10, 1973

Joseph A. Beirne sent a letter to me in which he said, "I note that eight of the eighteen members of the President's Committee have dissented in various respects over what is being proffered as the final report. Your statement and mine, however, were the only ones actually labeled as 'dissents.' We both make clear our great disappointment over the limited scope of the final report."

NOVEMBER 11, 1973

I had received several copies of the final report of the President's Committee on Health Education for distribution. Neither of my administrators, Mazur and Wehrle, responded to receiving the final report. USC President Hubbard sent a short letter thanking me for "bringing increased national visibility to our university."

I did receive many compliments on my dissent from leaders in the field. The following are a just a few examples of those statements:

"I thought your dissent was necessary and extremely lucid."
Herbert Jones
University of Maryland

"Your services on the President's Committee on Health Education brought a degree of professional acumen and personal dignity to that group that otherwise would have been conspicuously absent without you."
Robert S. Cobb
Mankato State College
Minnesota

"I really only wish to say that I support your point of view completely and that the comments by Victor Weingarten do not clarify but only tend to confuse and mislead the reader away from the key issues and arguments you present."
Donald C. McAfee
National Dairy Council

"You made your point, and I think you've done a tremendous job."
Morton A. Hill
Morality in Media, Inc.

"I was most pleased that you had the courage and commitment to dissent."
Michael C. Hosokawa
University of Oregon

"It took great courage to follow through with strong professional opinions. Keep up the good work."
Clifton O. Dummett, DDS
University of Southern California

"I received the President's Committee on Health Education Report. Congratulations on your bold and thoughtful dissent."
David B. Friedman, MD
Los Angeles County-USC Medical Center

"After having read your 'dissent,' I'm proud to know you."
Janet E. Burke, MPH
Department of Health
State of Minnesota

"I feel that the professionals in health education are proud of your stand."
Frank S. Stafford, MPH
Department of Health Services
County of Los Angeles

"I wish to express my appreciation to you for your formal dissent. Not only is it focused and relevant to the major weaknesses of the report, but you seem to be the only member whose views penetrated the consciousness of Director Weingarten at least to the extent that he was constrained to make a pitifully defensive comment."
Betty Mathews
University of Washington

Several times during my membership on the President's Committee, I had given serious thought to my involvement and the alternatives. Should I resign from the committee or allow myself to be a puppet? Standing alone really confronts the meaning of being an individual. I now know me—and I am not naive to the realities of the world around me. I carefully explored the consequences for believing and acting the way I did. I continued to stand for what I believed—so I could continue to live with myself.

Many of our young men and women in uniform have lost their lives for the freedom of dissent. A dissenter needs a lot of help from angels, family, friends, and mentors. I am thankful for them all.

APPENDIX

Excerpts from "The Report of the President's
Committee on Health Education."

The Report of the President's Committee on Health Education
801 Second Avenue
New York, New York 10017
212/889-6760

This information cited and the opinions expressed in this publication
are those of the President's Committee on Health Education and do
not necessarily reflect the views of the Health Services and Mental
Health Administration nor of the Department of Health, Education,
and Welfare.

A Comprehensive Health Education Program

In the final analysis, each individual bears the major responsibility for his own health. Unfortunately, too many of us fail to meet that responsibility. Too many Americans eat too much, drink too much, work too hard, and exercise too little. Too many are careless drivers.

These are personal questions, to be sure, but they are also public questions. For the whole society has a stake in the health of the individual. Ultimately, everyone shares in the cost of his illnesses or accidents. Through tax payments and through insurance premiums, the careful subsidize the careless; the non-smokers subsidize those who smoke; the physically fit subsidize the rundown and the overweight; the knowledgeable subsidize the ignorant and the vulnerable.

It is in the interest of our entire country, therefore, to educate and encourage each of our citizens to develop sensible health practices. Yet we have given remarkably little attention to the health education of our people.

Most of our current efforts in this area are fragmented and haphazard—a public service advertisement one week, a newspaper article another, a short lecture now and then from the doctor.

There is no national instrument, no central force to stimulate and coordinate a comprehensive health education program.

Richard Nixon
Health Message to Congress
February 15, 1971

Members of the President's Committee on Health Education

R. Heath Larry, chairman of the President's Committee on Health Education, is vice chairman of the board of directors of US Steel. Mr. Larry is a member of the National Commission on Productivity, appointed to that body by President Nixon, and a member of Governor Rockefeller's Steering Committee on Social Problems. He also serves as a board member of the Bituminous Coal Operators Association. He is a president of the Hospital Council of Western Pennsylvania and a trustee of Grove City College, the National YMCA Retirement Fund, and the US Council of the International Chamber of Commerce, Inc.

Walter J. McNerney, president of the Blue Cross Association, is vice chairman of the President's Committee on Health Education. He is president of the National Health Council; a member of the program committee of the Institute of Medicine, National Academy of Sciences; and president and chairman, Council of Management of the International Federation of Voluntary Health Service Funds. In 1970, Mr. McNerney served as chairman of HEW Secretary Finch's Task Force on Medicaid and Related Programs.

Joseph A. Beirne is president of the Communications Workers of America and a member of the executive council of the AFL-CIO, serving as chairman of its International Affairs Committee. He also is president of Postal, Telegraph, and Telephone International, secretary-treasurer of the American Institute for Free Labor Development, and a member of the National Commission on Productivity.

Leroy E. Burney, MD, is president of the Milbank Memorial Fund in New York City. Dr. Burney was appointed Surgeon General of the US Public Health Service by President Eisenhower in 1956 and served in that assignment until 1961. During that time, he also was chairman of the US delegation to the World Health Assembly and was its president in 1957. Dr. Burney is a former president of the National Health

Council and the Association of State and Territorial Health Officers, and president of the National Commission for the Study of Nursing and Nursing Education.

Joy G. Cauffman, PhD, is an associate professor in the School of Medicine at the University of Southern California. She has served as president or chairman of health-education associations on state, district, and national levels and currently is coordinator of the Coalition of National Health Education Organizations. Also, she currently is director of SEARCH: A Link to Services.

M. Alfred Haynes, MD, is chairman of the Department of Community Medicine and associate dean of the Charles R. Drew Postgraduate Medical School, Los Angeles, and chief of community medicine at the Martin Luther King Hospital in Los Angeles.

John Alexander McMahon is president of the American Hospital Association and former president of North Carolina Blue Cross and Blue Shield, Inc., in Durham and Chapel Hill, North Carolina. He is chairman of the board of trustees of Duke University; chairman of the Governor's Advisory Council on Comprehensive Health Planning, and former chairman, Health Planning Council for Central North Carolina, the state's first regional health planning agency; member, board of governors and executive committee of the Blue Cross Association; member, House of Delegates and Council on Financing, American Hospital Association; and member, Committee on the Health Services Industry, an advisory group to the agencies involved in Phase II of the Economic Stabilization Program.

A. C. Nielsen Jr. is president of A. C. Nielsen Company, an international market research organization. He is a member of the National Marketing Advisory Committee of the US Department of Commerce, the Presidential Advisory Council for Minority Enterprise, and the Peace Corps National Advisory Council, and serves as chairman of the Census Advisory Committee on Privacy and Confidentiality.

Joseph T. Painter, MD, practices internal medicine in the Ledbetter Clinic Association and is a Diplomate of the American Board of Internal Medicine. Dr. Painter is a past president of the American Society of Internal Medicine, having been a member of its board of trustees for six years, chairman of the Health Advisory Committee of the Texas State Office of Comprehensive Planning, and a member of the Medical Care Advisory committee of the Texas State Department of Welfare for Medicaid and of the board of directors for Blue Cross/ Blue Shield of Texas.

C. Wrede Petersmeyer is chairman and president of Corinthian Broadcasting Corporation and executive vice president and director of corporate planning and development of Dun & Bradstreet, Inc. He is a director of Dun & Bradstreet, Inc., and the Reuben H. Donnelley Corporation. He is a trustee of the Committee for Economic Development and is a member of its Research and Policy Committee. He is also a trustee of the Greenwich Savings Bank.

Dan Seymour is chairman and chief executive officer of the J. Walter Thompson Co. He was a member of the president's Council on Youth Opportunity and was the national communications coordinator of the council's summer programs. He is a member of the Ad Hoc Advisory Group on the Presidential Vote for Puerto Rico and a member of the Public Advisory Committee on Trade Policy, and a trustee and member of the executive committee of the Council of the Americas. He is also a director and member of the executive committee of the Boys' Clubs of America and a director of the American Association of Advertising Agencies.

Irving S. Shapiro, PhD, is director of the Health Education Division of the Health Insurance Plan of Greater New York. He holds faculty appointments at the Columbia School of Public Health, the Downstate

Medical School in Brooklyn, and Hunter College. He is a member of the Health Advisory Committee of the Public Affairs Committee, Inc., and of the New York State Board of Examiners for Nursing Home Administrators. He is a fellow of the American Public Health Association and of the Society of Public Health Education and is a member of the Association of Teachers of Preventive Medicine.

Charles A. Siegfried is vice chairman of the board and chairman of the executive committee of Metropolitan Life Insurance Company. He has served on HEW's Advisory Council on Social Security, on the Department of Labor's Advisory Council on Employee Welfare and Pension Benefit Plans, and as president of the Health Insurance Association of America. Currently, Mr. Siegfried is a director of the Anaconda Company and the Economic Development Council of New York City, chairman of the board of trustees of Franklin and Marshall College, and a member of the National Advisory Council of Opportunities Industrialization Centers of America.

Scott K. Simonds, DrPH, is a professor of health education and director of the Health Education Program at the University of Michigan School of Public Health. He is on the board of directors of the Epilepsy Foundation of America and is a member of the Advisory Committee on Community Health of the National Commission for the Study of Nursing and Nursing Education. Dr. Simonds is the immediate past president of the Society for Public Health Education and has served recently as consultant for the World Health Organization, the Pan American Health Organization, the US Public Health Service, the National Health Service Corps, and the White House Conference on Food, Nutrition, and Health.

J. Henry Smith is president of the Equitable Life Assurance Society in New York City and serves as a director of the Life Insurance Association of America and the Institute of Life Insurance. In addition, he is a member of the executive committee of the Association of New York State Life Insurance Companies. Mr. Smith has been chairman of the Health Insurance Council and is past president of the Health Insurance Association of America. He was appointed to the President's Commission on Income Maintenance Programs in 1968 and to the Governor's Advisory Commission on Social Concerns in 1970.

Ella Louise Strother is president of the Provident Comprehensive Neighborhood Health Council, Baltimore, and the executive vice president of Girl Scouts of Central Maryland. She also serves as a board member of the National Consumers Health Committee and was a member of the resident advisory board to the Commission of Housing and Urban Development.

Peggy Wright Wood is director of Public Health Social Work for the Onondaga County Department of Health in Syracuse, New York. She was formerly a member of the national advisory board for Planned Parenthood of America, the National Committee for Publications, Girl Scouts of America, Syracuse and Onondaga County, the Commission for Human Rights, and the Governor's Committee to Review New York Laws and Procedures in the Area of Human Rights. She is a member of the American Public Health Association, the New York State Public Health Association, and the National Association of Social Workers, Central New York Chapter.

Ex Officio

Richard P. McGrail has been deputy executive vice president of the American Cancer Society, Inc., since 1961 and has served the society in various capacities since 1946. A member of the New York County Lawyers Association and the Nassau Bar Association, Mr. McGrail is immediate past president of the National Health Council, and he now serves on its board.

Elliot Lee Richardson served as United States Secretary of Health, Education, and Welfare from June 6, 1970, until his confirmation as

Secretary of Defense in 1973. Prior to that, he was Under Secretary of State. From 1964 to 1966, as Lieutenant Governor of Massachusetts, he coordinated the state's health, education, and welfare programs and headed the task force that produced the Community Mental Health Act and developed a multiservice agency program. He was elected Attorney General of the Commonwealth in 1966. He is a former member of the board of overseers of Harvard College and is a member of the Council on Foreign Relations, a fellow of the American Academy of Arts and Sciences, and a fellow of the American Bar Foundation. He was appointed by President Nixon to the board of governors of the American National Red Cross.

Staff

Victor Weingarten, Director
Clarence E. Pearson, Associate Director
Linda Brannick, Staff Associate

Staff Assistants

Lynne Bernstein
Alvera Cleary
Carolyn Dutton
Josee Laventhol
Helene V. Malloy
Marion Sheshan
Laurel Stephens

Staff Council

Caesar Branchini
United Medical Services, Inc.
John Byrnes
Blue Cross of Greater New York

Howard Ennes
Equitable Life Assurance Society
Phyllis Ensor
The National Foundation—March of Dimes
Walter James
American Cancer Society
Robert Laur, PhD
US Department of Health, Education, and Welfare
Sol Lifson
National Tuberculosis and Respiratory Disease Association
Peter Meek
National Health Council
Levitte Mendel
National Health Council
Robert O'Connor, MD
US Steel Corporation
Diane Purseglove
National Health Council
Carl Rhodes
J. Walter Thompson
Justus Schifferers, PhD
Author
George M. Wheatley, MD
Metropolitan Life Insurance Company

Consultants

Milton Akers, EdD
Annie Butler, EdD
Pauline M. Carlyon
William Carlyon, PhD
Marjorie Craig
Roy Davis
Virginia Fernbach
Frank Ferro

Wallace Fulton
Edward D. Greenwood, MD
Peter Grevas
Mary J. Halstead
Marian Hamburg, EdD
Godfrey Hochbaum, PhD
Steven Homel, MD
Gertrude Hunter, MD
Anne E. Impellizzeri
Susan King-Hall
John P. Kirscht, PhD
Dell Kjer, PhD
David Klein, PhD
Lowell Levin
Elizabeth Mallory
Lawrence Mannuel, MD
Ann Nolte, PhD
Anne Pavlich
Bert Pence
Sam Raz
George Reader
Ruth Richards
Melvin Rudov, PhD
Elsa Schneider
John Senacor, EdD
Anna Skiff
Elena Sliepcevich, DPE
John Van Steenwyck
Kathy Toland
Matisyohu Weisenberg, PhD
Alexander Williams

Letter of Transmittal

Dear Mr. President:

Your Committee on Health Education has completed the assignment you gave it September 14, 1971. On behalf of the committee, I thank you for making it possible for those of us on the committee to discover for ourselves—and hopefully, through this report, for the benefit of the nation—how deplorably this country is neglecting a vast opportunity to help people help themselves to have better health.

The recent and continuing debate over national health insurance has uncovered a great deal of concern about the delivery and financing of health care. That concern is felt by the public as well as by government and private institutions both inside and outside of the health field.

However, after more than a year of intensive study and research, we are convinced that results of any changes or improvements in the delivery and financing of health care will be virtually nullified unless there is, at the same time, an improvement in health education—which means not just supplying information about health to people, but motivating them to accept the information and put it to work in their daily lives.

Unfortunately, the important, and often crucial role the individual can play in maintaining his own health has rarely been clearly explained or adequately dramatized.

Our findings regarding the ignorance or apathy—or both—of American institutions and organizations, indeed, the public at large, toward health education are chronicled in the body of our report. A few of the major findings can, however, be summarized in a few paragraphs:

- While the need and demand for health-care services have been rising, health education has been neglected. Many, perhaps most major causes of sickness and death can be affected—and some prevented—by individual behavior, yet the whole field of health education is fragmented, uneven in effectiveness, and lacks any base of operations. No agency inside or outside of government is either responsible for, or even assists in setting goals, maintaining criteria of performance, or measuring results.

- School health education in most primary and secondary schools is either not provided at all or is tacked onto other subject matter such as physical education or biology, assigned to teachers whose main interests and qualifications lie elsewhere.

- In many states, legislation actually impedes development of effective school health programs. Some state laws regarding what can be taught have not been changed since the late 1800s.

- The US Office of Education (Department of HEW), in a report prepared for the committee, could not cite a single program of research or evaluation it is supporting in the area of school health education.

- What is taught to children is not made meaningful enough to stay with them. Nutrition studies show that teenagers— especially girls—often damage their health through poor eating habits. Other studies show that youngsters who once urged their parents not to smoke have themselves become cigarette smokers as teenagers.

- For all age groups, health education has generally been stereotyped. Its programs have not been—but must be— structured to reflect the cultural mores of each population group being approached. There is vital need for innovation and experimentation with new kinds of educational programs.

- The vast majority of people—88 percent in one population survey—look to their physicians or TV commercials for information about health. Yet evidence presented to the committee indicates that physicians are often too busy to do an effective job, and too many TV messages are primarily concerned with product promotion rather than with true consumer health education. Providers of care, such as hospitals, do little to overcome deficiencies. Neither voluntary health organizations nor insurance carriers (private or nonprofit) have exploited fully their opportunities.

- Of $75 billion spent last year for medical, hospital, and health care—more than $200 million a day—about 92 percent is spent for treatment after illness occurs. Of the remaining amount, more than half is spent for biomedical research. Prevention of illness and health education share the balance, with health education receiving the short end.

- Of $18.2 billion allocated in 1973 for medical and health activities of the Department of HEW, only $30 million is for specific programs in health education; $14 million more for general programs. That amounts to less than one-fourth of 1 percent. Of $7.3 billion allocated for health purposes to all other federal agencies, even a smaller fraction is spent on health education.

- On the state level, health departments spend less than half of 1 percent of their budgets for health education.

- A considerable number of employers have become concerned with acute, dramatic, work-related problems, such as alcohol and drug abuse. But business, industry, and labor are not significantly involved in overall programs that could contribute to sound off-job safety and health practices that could also benefit on-job attendance and productivity.

As you will see in the report, it is evident from our inquiry that the needs, problems, and opportunities in health education are so large, so urgent, and so complex that progress will depend upon a major long-term commitment to it by the nation's leaders.

It is equally evident that the responsibility, the challenge, and the burden of providing for the widespread need, solving the problems, and meeting the opportunities must be shared by all concerned and capable parties in both the public and private sectors of society.

To bring public and private efforts together, and to provide a focal point for the nation's multiple health-education activities, the committee has recommended establishment of a "National Center for Health Education" to be authorized by the Congress and sustained by both public and private support.

In addition, we have developed a list of additional recommendations—for governmental and private activities—to develop, strengthen, unify, and evaluate health education in this nation. Details will be found in the four sections of the report:

1. "Changing Needs for Health Education," describing changes in health problems and the methods of health care in the last few decades and pointing out their implications for health education.
2. "Purposes and Challenges of Health Education," showing what health education is and what it can hope to do.
3. "National Activities in Support of Health Education," telling how virtually every element of society can play a role in making health education a reality.
4. "National Center for Health Education," proposing the establishment of a central organization to stimulate and coordinate effective programs in health education.

It is important to note that while our subject is health education, we have tried to stress throughout the report that substantial improvement in the health of Americans depends on many factors outside of the medical structure as well as on those inside it. Certainly there is a need to work with the whole health-care delivery system to assure that every person has access to it and that every person who enters the system benefits from it to the highest extent possible. But at the same time, we must recognize that good health also is affected by broader opportunities for good jobs, a reduction in joblessness and its consequent poverty, more adequate housing, a higher level of education, and an upgrading of the physical environment.

I particularly appreciate the degree to which consensus became possible—notwithstanding that each individual brought to the committee's deliberation a separate and distinct background of experience—which led almost to as many separate and distinct views concerning what should become the major emphasis of the report. As is inevitable, some viewpoints are expressed with less emphasis than some members would feel appropriate. Hence, this document may share some of the shortcomings that so often must characterize the product of committees. Nevertheless, we are hopeful that what has emerged—for the most part as our consensus—will contribute to the ongoing emphasis upon health education—upon the importance of which we are totally unanimous.

As a final thought, on my behalf, I would like to express my special appreciation to the agencies, organizations, and institutions whose executives, staff, or faculty were given the time and support to serve on the committee. The dedication of each committee member, and the time each gave to the work of the committee, are the ultimate assets that made this report possible.

Sincerely yours,
R. Heath Larry
Chairman

Charge to the Committee

1. To *describe* the "state of the art" in health education of the public in the United States today by means of broad-sweep inquiries that would:
   (a) *Identify* the principal areas of activity; the institutions, agencies, programs involved; the characteristics of programs and ongoing activities; the interrelationships and interdependencies of the activities; and
   (b) *Assess* effectiveness and levels of participation in terms of the principal component function of health education of the public, with particular reference to behavioral change and community action.
2. To *define* the nation's need for health-education programs and their basic characteristics, in terms of major groupings of health consumers, including the well and the nonwell; mothers, children, and youths; the working population; residents of the inner cities and rural areas; the aged; and the disabled.
3. To *establish* goals, priorities, and immediate and long-range objectives of a comprehensive, nationwide effort to raise the level of "health consumer citizenship."
4. To *propose* the most appropriate scope, function, structure, organization, and financing of such an effort, possibly in the form of a "National Health Education Foundation," giving particular attention to constructive activities now performed by private, professional, and governmental groups.
5. To *develop* a plan for the implementation of its recommendations.

The Scope of Health Education of the Public

The term "health education of the public"—*consumer health education*—embraces those processes of communication and education that help each individual learn how to achieve and maintain a reasonable level of health appropriate to his particular needs and interests, and to be motivated to follow personal and community health practices that contribute to his state of health and well-being—a positive concept going well beyond the mere absence of disease or infirmity.

The Health Consumer Education that this committee is asked to facilitate for the nation is a process that could dynamically involve the entire citizenry, and should be oriented toward individual and community action. The focus should be on the whole person in his natural community, and on the individual's needs and responsibilities:

- first, to *know* himself, and to shape his lifestyle to maximize his personal options for living fully
- second, to *utilize* health resources and services and environmental support, with optimal efficiency and economy
- third, to *participate* constructively in community health and environmental planning, in priority setting, and in decision making

Consequently, the deliberation of this committee should encompass the full range of elements that go into this broad concept of *health consumer citizenship*. The committee's inquiries would probe into such factors as disease, disability, and accident prevention … the health care in hospitals, health maintenance organizations, and other health facilities and systems … public health, and environmental health, and human ecological consideration … exercise, diet, and nutrition … rehabilitation … mental health … educational programs and educational aspects of health services in schools, in day-care facilities, in industries, and on farms—and their interrelationships with other community health activities … recruiting, training, and career development of health personnel, both those needed for health consumer education services and those concerned with delivery of health care ... techniques of communication, including the mass media, electronics and audiovisual systems, health museums ... research and development in social and behavioral fields, technology, and community organizations.

Activities of the Committee

To do its job, the committee:

1. Held eight public hearings in major cities, at which seventy-one hours of testimony were taken from almost three hundred persons from forty-seven states and Puerto Rico. Witnesses represented groups and organizations in both the private and public sectors that were doing effective health-education work or who had knowledge of the region's health-education needs.

2. Met with directors of twenty-two neighborhood health centers from various parts of the country to learn what they had found out about health education through their work with low-income families and individuals.

3. Asked six hundred producers of health-education materials and programs to list on a questionnaire their most effective programs as well as their greatest disappointments—plus their view of priorities in health education.

4. Appointed special subcommittees to work directly with business and labor groups, prepayment plans and private insurance companies, professional associations, voluntary health agencies, philanthropic foundations, school health agencies, government, and mass media.

5. Commissioned papers from authorities on such subjects as motivation and behavior; school health; educational opportunities in group practice units; health-education programs in hospitals; and cost effectiveness of health-education programs in industry.

6. Met with twenty-seven federal agencies to determine the potential health-education role of government as a major employer.

7. Examined the experience of the British Health Education Foundation and met with representatives of more than twenty

countries through the World Health Organization to find out what they were doing that would benefit this study.

8. Convened special conferences of experts in such fields as school health education, motivation and behavior, and mass media to discuss key issues in health education.

9. Solicited and received written statements and reports from scores of informed individuals and organizations setting forth their views of health-education problems and priorities.

10. Distributed more than fifteen thousand copies of a brochure describing the mission of the committee and soliciting information and knowledge that would assist the committee in its work.

11. Through the auspices of the National Health Council, which devoted its 1972 National Health Forum to the work of the committee, met with the approximately six hundred participants over two days to explore their points of view as to directions the committee should take in its work.

12. Committee members and staff met and spoke to a variety of professional organizations and societies, among them the American Medical Association, American Nurses Association, American Public Health Association, American Hospital Association, etc., describing the work of the committee and soliciting information that would be useful to it in its deliberations.

Supplementary Statements

M. Alfred Haynes, MD
Chairman
Department of Community Medicine
Charles R. Drew Postgraduate Medical School

I cannot endorse the recommendation of an operating budget of $12–15 million for the national center even over a period of five years without at the same time insisting on accountability to the public. The expenditure of this amount may not be enough to do the job that has to be done, but it may be too much for what the center may actually accomplish. One way of determining this is to hold the center firmly responsible to the public. The committee, as a whole, has been timid about making this recommendation because it does not know a perfect way to do so. Even an imperfect method of ensuring accountability may be better than none at all if that method carries with it the flexibility to permit change. Furthermore, the element of public accountability could prove to be one of the most effective health-education techniques that the center could devise.

I propose that the center be made accountable to a number of provider organizations, such as the National Health Council and the Coalition of Health Educators, and also a number of consumer organizations, such as the National Consumer Health Organization and the National Chicano Health Organization. After a reasonable period of time, such as three years, and periodically thereafter, the center would be under obligation to report to these organizations exactly what it has done and with what results. It is possible that the center could generate so little interest that no organization could care whether it really existed. In that case, it should die a quiet and natural death or be painlessly defunded. If, on the other hand, its accomplishments were such as to justify additional expenditure of funds, these organizations should not only endorse but contribute financially to its support.

Inherent in this approach is the risk that the center may not survive, but then no organization should survive if its performance does not merit survival.

Richard P. McGrail
Deputy Executive Vice President
American Cancer Society

I think the definition of health education could be strengthened. It might read somewhat as follows:

1. Health education is a planned process focusing on involvement of both health worker and consumer in its planning and implementation. Learning and behavior are facilitated through the two-way communication of information, knowledge, values, and attitudes.
2. We may be somewhat prejudiced, but cigarette smoking is given very light treatment as a problem; we believe it should have been listed as one of the major health problems in the report.

C. Wrede Petersmeyer
Chairman and President
Corinthian Broadcasting Corp.

I believe that the center should carry the responsibility for preparing creative, persuasive health information promotional spots for television and radio; advertisements for newspapers, magazines, outdoor and transportation displays; and literature for distribution through health agencies, companies, and governmental offices. The center should then be able to arrange with stations to carry such spots and with the print and display media to carry such advertisements in the public interest and without charge. In order to carry out this responsibility, the center's staff should include as a key executive a professional, experienced communicator. To assist him in his duties, he could mobilize the services, on a volunteer basis, of a task force of the best creative talent in the private and public sector.

Irving S. Shapiro, PhD
Director, Health Education Division
Health Insurance Plan of Greater New York

I am in full accord with the bulk of the report and particularly with the major recommendation that a National Center for Health Education of the Public be established. I do dissent from several important statements and views in the report, as follows:

1. In Section II, "Purposes and Challenges of Health Education," the fact that health education has been fragmented and largely unevaluated is cited as resulting in a health-care system overburdened with patients because of their lack of knowledge. If indeed our health-care "system" is "overburdened," to blame it on patients who presumably would not be patients if only they had learned to behave more wisely is unacceptable and astonishing. It is far more likely that there is inefficiency because the system itself is fragmented and unevaluated.

    The same acceptable attitude is expressed in the statement shortly thereafter that people must meet the health-care delivery system "at least halfway." The presumption here is that they are equally, if not more, to blame for the failures in our "system."

    The final expression of this unacceptable view is contained in the report statement that those served by the "providers of health care" share an obligation with them for "making a total health-care system work." No reference is made to the role the consumer or citizen should play in determining the nature and shape of the "system" itself. Perhaps his responsibility is *not* to make the available "system" work, but to change it first!

2. In the section "Habit and Attitude Changes," it is stated
    that violations of common sense, such as cigarette smoking,
    faulty diet, and drug abuse "represent a major weakness in the
    nation's past health-education efforts." Since the burden of the
    report, correctly, is that health education in contradistinction
    to factual exhortations, appeals, and warnings, has not been
    adequately supported and tested. It may appear disingenuous
    to fault health education for the weakness inherent in the
    sole or major reliance on information packaging and delivery
    which characterizes the very situation we seek to change.

3. In the section "Environmental Protection," responsibility for
    pollution is assigned to "all of society." Yet only the public
    and industry are specified for the task of sharing in the costs
    and solution efforts. This, I feel, is a distortion of particular
    importance in view of the overwhelming threats to health
    that environmental pollution poses. The major force for
    achieving a clean, healthy environment in this country is
    government, on the national, state, and local levels, and in
    both the legislative and executive branches.

    This section as it stands, in a report on health education,
    clearly implies that if the public is educated to bear their share
    of the cost, industry will cut their pollution of the rivers, reduce
    undue noise, redesign goods and materials, and install smoke-
    abatement mechanisms. As experience demonstrates, and as
    the regional nature of the major pollution problems demands,
    only governmental standards, controls, enforcement, and
    financial participation can truly begin to protect the public
    health from environmental hazards.

Charles A. Siegfried
Vice Chairman of the Board
Metropolitan Life Insurance Company

A number of aspects of the report cause me to wish to indicate
certain of my concerns and reservations. On the one hand, the report

appears to minimize both the volume and quality of what has been done and is being done in the way of health education. On the other hand, it tends to minimize the enormous complexities in the way of making significant changes. Numerous recommendations are made for extensive new activities without any clear indication of just what they might accomplish, what they would likely cost, or whether the hoped-for improvements would be commensurate with the costs.

A major recommendation is that there be created a National Center for Health Education. Not only do I think it desirable to have more information than we currently have available as to the sources of funds and the operational relationships of the proposed organization, but I think more thought should be given to the nature and significance of the research, which is envisaged as an important function and which would be designed "to find ways to persuade people of different lifestyles to modify those styles in order to contribute to the quality of their lives."

Despite the great amount of commendable effort that has gone into the report, the vastness of the material and the importance of the subject strongly indicate the need for more deliberation before action programs can appropriately be recommended or new institutions be established.

Scott K. Simonds, DrPH
Professor of Health Education
School of Public Health
University of Michigan

The opportunity to make a statement of dissent is appreciated; however, I prefer to write a "statement of conscience" rather than a statement of dissent to be included in the report. With the exception of the specific recommendation mentioned below, I can accept most of the report. I know that this tenth and final draft represents a synthesis of a great deal of information and a compromise of many opinions from members of the committee and from the many people throughout the country who participated in our work. In consolidating information in the several drafts of the report, however, some of the most interesting and significant ideas have been lost that described ways in which health education could be advanced in this country. I think this is to be regretted.

As chairman of the Committee on Education, which focused its attention on health education of preschool and school-age children and college youths, I feel strongly that a wealth of testimony and expert opinion that we obtained in our committee has surfaced only as the tip of an iceberg in the final report. Some of the substantive contributions have been lost entirely. Although much information must be condensed in a report of this kind, I do hope that the really important material brought together for the committee can be utilized to support the work of the many community leaders and professionals in health education who have labored long and hard to achieve a higher quality of health education for the children and youth of this country, to whom we are ultimately accountable, and to set the stage for changes in social policy at the national level.

I am forced to dissent from the recommendation at the bottom of page 28 of the present copy primarily because of its wording and hence its implications. It reads, "Is recommended that schools of medicine, health science, and public health cooperate with schools of education to qualify administrators and teachers to perform and administer health-education programs. Since every health-education program cannot be run by a professional health educator, serious consideration should be given to preparing selected persons as 'paramedics,' in effect, in the field of health education."

First of all, it is not at all clear who the administrators are who are referred to in this statement. Administrators of community health-education programs are already prepared in schools of public health and other programs accredited by the American Public Health Association. If school administrators are the focus, which I believe is the intent, then the sentence should so state. The phrase "to perform" implies "to perform health-education programs," and the meaning is, therefore, not clear. I think the phrase "since every health-education program cannot be run by a professional health educator" begs the question. There is a need for adequate training funds and funded positions to assure that as many programs in the community and in the schools as possible are indeed directed by professionally trained health educators. There is also a need, however, for health-education aides, and much progress has already been made to define their roles and functions and to employ them in community health-education programs. Their tasks are not administrative as implied in this recommendation, however, nor are they "paramedics" in any sense of the word. In my opinion they are "para-educs" if such a distinction is necessary.

In closing, I think it is regrettable that the name of the proposed national center has been shortened in this report from earlier versions to Center for Health Education without the designation that the public is to be the major focus of its attention. The problems that will arise through misinterpretation of the functions of the organization will be considerable. It will be assumed by many that the education of health manpower is the focus from the title alone when, indeed, it was our intent to direct attention to health education of the public.

J. Henry Smith
President
The Equitable Life Assurance Society

The basic theme of this committee report is that health education of the public must be made more complete and effective if this nation is to achieve optimal improvement in its health status. That position seems unassailable. Furthermore, I agree that a broadly based "national center," as a focal point of action and a catalyst, could effectively promote health education.

However, under the constraints of time and funding, the committee was unable to deal in depth with the problems of health education and with the complexities and interrelationships involved in the concept of the "national center." Consequently, I remain uneasy about this report in two respects.

First, there is a need for further clarification and development of the concept of the proposed center. Certainly before it can be expressed in legislative form, there will have to be extensive development of such questions as to how the center will relate to other agencies, institutions, and the government; how it will be financed in detail; and the process by which it will be held accountable to the American public.

Second, in an attempt to identify the realities of health education, this report makes a myriad of specific recommendations. While many of these are important and probably valid, again, within the constraints on the committee, a number of the recommendations seem to me to be somewhat cursory. Some of them overlook the well-documented warning of the report itself that the serious difficulties in health education include not only the dissemination of information but motivating people to use the information wisely. It would have been better, it seems to me, to have relegated the various problems to the proposed center for attention. The center, with careful study, experimentation, and cooperative effort among the many groups concerned, should produce more valid and productive recommendations, and stimulate development of more effective programs, than our committee was able to do in its lifespan.

Ella L. Strother
Provident Comprehensive Neighborhood Health Center
Baltimore, Maryland

Having examined and deliberated at great length over the final report of the President's Committee on Health Education, I find that I cannot support or approve the complete report. Therefore, I support the report only with reservations. While there is much in the report that I do support, my primary concern involves those parts that are inaccurate or misleading. Among them are:

> (1) The implication that the entire committee rejected
> the idea that the Departments of HEW-OEO could

not do the work as proposed for the new foundation. I do not and have not concurred in that decision.

(2) The report mentions meeting with the directors of neighborhood health centers, but it does not state that these directors made a special plea that the government extend the life of OEO and that the funds and purposes of HEW-OEO would not be eliminated or diluted. This same appeal has been made by the poor and near-poor people throughout the country. Yet the report has ignored this appeal and the harm, both mentally and physically, to the poor and near poor, which is already being done and which can be greatly increased by diverting both funds and functions of HEW-OEO.

While the report mentions manpower, it lacks substantial substance and direction. There was insufficient information on the effect of low income and insufficient jobs for people who want to work. It is my position that the position of the lady who stated in effect, before the committee "that she did not need anyone to tell her how to cook or what to cook, what she needed was a good job so she could buy what she knew she needed" reflects the opinion and plea of many. Third, the committee's report does not do justice to the work and accomplishments of the Departments of HEW-OEO in elevating both the health and health education of the people in the community. The truth is practically all of the recommendations made in the report are being executed in OEO- and perhaps HEW-funded health centers. The main weakness of HEW-OEO to date is the lack of coordination. If any program is going to be accountable to the people rather than directed to the people, then the people, like institutions, must be given a reasonable time to organize.

The accountability of a national health center is lacking in the report. Many consumers have stated that federally funded health programs should be accountable to the people they propose to serve.

I concur with that conclusion. If a national health center for health education is to serve the American public, it should be accountable to the American people—and it should have more than token representation from the poor and near-poor members of our society at every level of policy and decision making that affects them.

While some of the issues of "dissent" concerning the report of the President's Committee on Health Education as expressed by Dr. Joy G. Cauffman may not be completely obvious in the report, it is my opinion that the items of "dissent" have validity, and it is unfortunate that greater attention was not paid to them.

Dissents

Joseph A. Beirne
President
Communications Workers of America, AFL-CIO

If the President's Committee on Health Education presents the proposed report to the president, I believe we will have missed, or at least delayed for a considerable time, an opportunity to change public attitudes toward health. It is with reluctance that I dissent from this report.

We already have lost five years. In late 1967, the National Advisory Commission on Health Manpower made recommendations on the kind of consumer-oriented health education envisioned by President Nixon when he formed the present committee. I do not believe we will be doing the president a service by proffering this report, since Mr. Nixon showed so great an interest in health education in his Health Message to the Congress of February 15, 1971, and in his subsequent charge to the committee.

The report, as presented for final ratification by members of the committee, also does an injustice to the nearly three hundred citizens and health professionals who testified at the eight public hearings, in my view.

I strongly believe that the National Center for Health Education, if formed within the framework of this report, will not be effective. And thus, in the future, it will be doubly difficult to do a proper job because of a need to undo what has been improperly entered upon. I do not agree with the first sentence of the letter of transmittal that the committee has completed its work, and I will explain briefly below.

In the letter of transmittal, the committee would note that only $30 million is allocated in fiscal 1973 for specific programs in health education, plus $14 million for general programs, both within the budget of the Department of Health, Education, and Welfare. To that total of $44 million would be added up to $3 million a year, according to the final paragraph of Section IV, "Findings and Recommendations:

National Center for Health Education." Thus, the letter of transmittal and Section IV tell the president that less than twenty-five cents per person per year is envisioned for health-education purposes. If we of the committee attempt to tell the president that the proposed amounts will have an effect on health education, we will be doing a disservice to the nation. Other portions of the proposed report, especially Section II, describe a sizeable problem.

Section III proposes a private, nonprofit organization with a congressional mandate, financed jointly by federal and private funds. The Corporation for Public Broadcasting, established on those lines, for nearly five years has proven unable to function because of the tangled relationship between those two basic sources of funds.

The central entity, which would serve as catalyst and "gadfly," is the only logical means of achieving what we have—altogether too timidly in this report—seen is necessary. It will achieve only if the needed funds and personal and organizational commitments are present.

In Section IV, I note that the center would be a source of information and expertise for lawmakers, but it would not lobby on its own behalf for the necessary authorization and appropriations. Since the proposed report does not state who will be the advocate in the legislative process, there is the strong possibility that there will be no advocate. Anyone who has had any connection with the legislative process in Washington is aware that a socially useful program must have strong advocates to go beyond the mere idea stage. The lack of definitive information—for which I have asked since May 1972—as to the degree of commitment from the professional health organizations leads me to the conclusion that that commitment is nonexistent. It is impossible to find, anywhere in this draft report, the mere mention of the chief professional health organizations; nor is it possible to find definitive information as to what the special subcommittee was able to achieve with the professional groups. Four of these groups are key to success: American Medical Association, American Hospital Association, American Public Health Association, and American Dental Association. For our report to have meaning, I believe we should be able to tell the president that these have joined in the efforts of the President's Committee on Health Education.

When in May 1972 I forwarded preliminary views on the committee's work, I believed the committee was not confronting the issues head-on. I do not see that situation changed in the final draft.

Joy G. Cauffman, PhD
School of Medicine
University of Southern California

Having had such great faith and expectations in the work of the President's Committee on Health Education, it is with keen disappointment that I find it necessary to dissent from the report to the president. My professional ethics and integrity, however, offer me no alternative. In preparing this dissent, my goal has been to state the facts as I see them, and when possible, to offer constructive suggestions that will prove useful to individuals and groups who are interested in improving the quality of life and the health of the nation through health education.

Goals Left Unfulfilled

A careful analysis of the report clearly demonstrates that the goals set forth in the president's charge to the committee and held forth to the general public were never fully achieved by the committee.

Committee Procedures Irregular

The report represents the end product of over a year's work by the committee. Efforts leading to the report were conducted under conditions in which staff was permitted to usurp committee responsibility and in which committee leadership was ineffective in pursuing the president's assignment. Processes involved in producing the report have not contributed to its credibility. For example, information submitted to the staff often either never reached or was censored before reaching the full committee. Committee leadership involved its members in meaningless exercises and failed to properly use their talents and resources.

The Nature and Meaning of Health Education Distorted

The substance of the report becomes distorted because of its failure to clearly focus on the subject of health education. Obviously, health education should be the central issue since both the title of the committee and the charge to the committee explicitly state this responsibility. However, the report improperly emphasizes ancillary issues, such as the history of medicine and public health, health problems, and health care. In the process of interweaving health education with other ancillary issues, essential distinctions are not always clearly delineated and viable linkages are not always provided between the ancillary issues and health education. Thus, the total conceptualization of the report lacks rational thinking, continuity, suitable perspective, and integration. Because of these significant deficiencies in the report, the nature and meaning of health education are heavily clouded and the report becomes less than professional in its misdirected effort to interpret health education to the public.

Leadership Opportunities for Professional Health Educators Denied

The report does not provide the leadership opportunities that professional health educators rightfully deserve and are capable of assuming. The change to remove any prejudicial barrier that may stand between their professional capability and achievement is lost. For example, the report should, but does not, specify that the National Center for Health Education will have both an administrator and a health-education director. The director should be a professional health educator with a background and experience in community and school health education and should hold a position in the center that is analogous to a position held by a physician who is a medical director in a hospital. Further, the report should, but does not, specify that professional community and school health educators should share leadership roles for health education at high policy-making and administrative levels within federal, state, and local government.

Support for Critical Health-Educator Manpower Shortages Omitted

The report reflects the need for increased health-educator manpower in the United States, particularly in early childhood, school, and hospital settings. At the same time, the report fails to recommend support of training programs for professional health educators, but it conversely recommends support of training programs for nonprofessionals, such as "paramedics" and volunteers who are to perform health-education functions. Extending nonprofessional manpower in health education without proportionate expansions in already depleted professional health-educator ranks places an unrealistic burden on existing manpower. Therefore, the federal government should, as a manpower priority, extend its present training programs for community health educators to include school health educators. The more than one hundred institutions of higher education in the United States that prepare professional health educators and that are capable of contributing a strong basic health science input should conduct these training programs.

The Unified Voice for the Health-Education Profession Ignored

The report discriminates against the Coalition of National Health Education Organizations[1] representing the unified voice of the health-education profession and consisting of all national health-education organizations in the United States with identifiable health-educator memberships and ongoing health-education programs. This is apparent since only a single reference is made to the coalition in the

---

1 Member organizations of the coalition include the American Association for Health, Physical Education, and Recreation, School Health Division; the American College Health Association, Health Education Section; the American Public Health Association, Public Health Education Section and School Health Section; the American School Health Association, the Conference of State and Territorial Directors of Public Health Education; the Society of State Directors of Health, Physical Education, and Recreation; and the Society for Public Health Education, Inc.

table of organization for the National Center for Health Education. This single reference clearly shows that the coalition would have no direct role in establishing center policy. In an effort that anticipates mounting a comprehensive nationwide health-education program, it is inconceivable that the primary full-time providers of health-education services in this country are virtually ignored. Thwarting the profession dissipates valuable trained resources contributing to the nation's health. As a result, the American people stand to lose.

Value of Mass Media Not Fully Recognized

While no health-education program can be fully and effectively implemented through only mass media, it would have been important for the report to clearly specify the dimensions of mass media's involvement since media have potential for both favorably and unfavorably influencing the quality of life for millions of Americans. The report does pay passing attention to the subject of mass media in relation to the National Center for Health Education, but it otherwise neglects to encourage sound linkages between health-education practitioners and mass media specialists within both large networks and local outlets.

National Center for Health Education
Unaccountable to the Nation

The report projects "the operating budget of the center for the first five years would be $12 million to $15 million" and "The program budget would be somewhat higher." The budget projections however do not specify major categories of anticipated expenditures and do not relate expenditures to functions of the center. Therefore, specifications of functional priorities within the center have not been delineated within the report. In addition, the report also fails to develop a plan of evaluation, including accountability for center functions. Such an omission is particularly difficult to understand in the light of the numerous findings and recommendations on the subject of evaluation within the report, and in view of the role the center will play in evaluating the health-education efforts of others. If clearly described evaluation programs apply to all other health-education programs, the center should not be immune; to the contrary, the center is to serve the American public—it must be accountable to the people. To do otherwise is hypocrisy.

American People, Victims of False Promises

All who wished to testify at the regional hearings held in major cities across the nation during January 1972 were given an opportunity to be heard. Many speakers waited endless hours to testify and were promised that their presentations would be given careful attention. It is a grievous fault that the full committee never reviewed the total input in recorded form or through a carefully prepared summary. This casual treatment of information by the committee demonstrates its failure to utilize the full range of information received in selecting major ideas for the report.

Following the National Health Forum, which was held in New Orleans in March 1972, *Medical World News* reported that the committee did not keep its promise to participants by providing preliminary findings at the forum. This was true. Participants at the forum, however, were assured by committee leadership that their input would be carefully considered by the full committee. This was not done. Even more distressing is the fact that the body of the report does not even mention the National Health Forum.

Implementation and Follow-up Disregarded

The report includes more than thirty recommendations under the label of "National Activities in Support of Health Education." The fact is that many of the recommendations address themselves to responsibilities that should be carried out by or in cooperation with state and local leadership. In addition, supportive evidence to clarify the recommendations and to make implementation readily feasible is missing from the report. As examples, the report recommends that model laws for school health-education programs be encouraged, but it fails to suggest content to be included in such laws; the report further recommends that the nation's hospitals provide health-education programs, but it fails to suggest the nature and scope of such programs. The report should contain guidelines for immediate action and follow-up of the report at community, state, and national levels, and it should provide a blueprint for future planning and action associated with a comprehensive nationwide health-education effort.